GUT
HEALTH
SECRETS
— *for* —
WOMEN

Proven **Diet** And **Stress Reduction**
Strategies To Enhance Your
Digestive Health, Balance
Hormones And **Feel Better** Than Ever

NAOMI OLSON

ISBN: 978-1-915217-31-8 (paperback)

Scan the QR code below to get your free copy of the 4-week gut health reset plan!

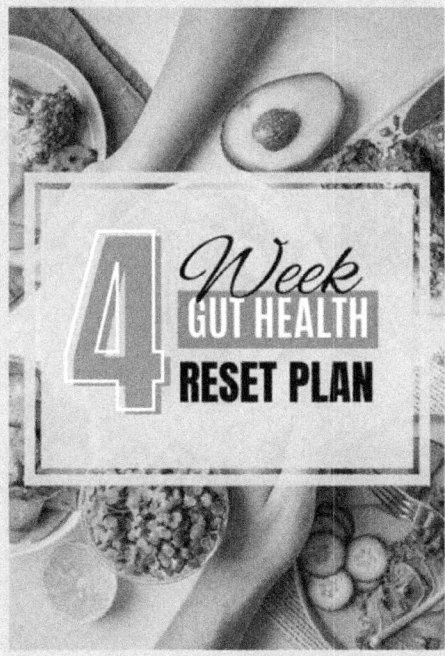

Table of Contents

Introduction 6

Chapter 1 A Closer Look Inside Your Gut...10

Chapter 2 The Importance of Microbiota 18

Chapter 3 The Most Common Gut Problems...30

Chapter 4 Signs, Causes and Effects of Poor Gut Health 39

Chapter 5 Food Intolerances 52

Chapter 6 Detox and Reset.. 88

Chapter 7 Heal and Nourish the Gut..100

Chapter 8 Retaining Good Long-Term Gut Health Through Diet............112

Chapter 9 Stress and Self-Care...123

Chapter 10 The Importance of Moving Your Body and Getting Good Sleep........136

Conclusion 160

Glossary...163

Bibliography 167

Introduction

"The road to health is paved with good intestines!" – Sherry A. Rogers (an internationally recognized expert in medicine).

I want to start this book with a little story about one of my best friends. She had organized a great trip to Paris. There were lots of things to do, and not a lot of time to do them, but she set off to see *all* the sights, on a packed schedule. She went up the Eiffel Tower, she visited Notre Dame, she saw the Arc de Triomphe and the Champs Elysees, and then she went to the Louvre... and she was really looking forward to seeing the Mona Lisa, but she suddenly realized she *needed* to find the bathroom, and fast.

Fortunately, she made it in time – but she never got to see the Mona Lisa. Time was too short!

Maybe you've had that kind of experience, or maybe you're just used to putting up with low-level nuisances like nausea, constipation, acid reflux, heartburn, bloatedness, or gas. There are all kinds of ways your gut will let you know it's not happy, and it can make your life really miserable. So this book will look at ways you can keep your gut healthy and happy, and make your life much easier!

The gut isn't given much respect, but it's one of the most important organs in your body. The gastrointestinal tract develops rapidly in the first three months or so of your life, and when you reach adulthood it contains somewhere round about 100 trillion microorganisms or microbiota. These work together to help your body absorb nutrients and process waste.

But your gut does other things that it's not often given credit for. For instance, it links to your immune system; about three-quarters of the body's immune cells are located in the gut. If you're always catching colds, maybe it's your gut that's getting you down!

The gut also affects your feelings and mood. Your enteric nervous system has so many neurotransmitters, it's practically a 'second brain.'

The story of the gut starts dramatically. A baby's stomach triples in size in just its first three days of life. And from birth to the age of five, the small intestine doubles in length. That's really fast growth and it's accompanied by the development of the whole digestive system – different enzymes, new functions, and biochemical processes.

During this time, all kinds of events can affect this development: the type of birth, whether a baby was born prematurely, the mother's diet during pregnancy or breastfeeding, the kind of nutrition the child receives, and the use of antibiotics in the early years (which can kill off many of the beneficial microbes in the gut, as well as the bad ones they're meant to exterminate). Imbalances in the gut related to childhood deficiencies can be linked to increases in the prevalence of asthma, allergies, and colic.

The impact can take a heavy toll on your life. Bad gut health can increase your chances of having Crohn's disease, ulcerative colitis, or IBS (irritable bowel syndrome). Some kinds of bacteria can increase your cholesterol levels, or your chances of kidney disease, because they create a chemical that your liver turns to trimethylamine-N-oxide (TMAO), and this leads to cholesterol build-up. Or your gut neurotransmitters can make you feel hungry when you're actually full. Guess what? That can end up making you obese.

Women need to be careful, since IBS is twice as common in women than in men. It also makes women feel a whole lot worse, and they can experience much more fatigue, depression, and anxiety as a result than men usually do.

I know this from experience. I've suffered from IBS all my working life. At first, I thought there was nothing I could do about it. I didn't really want to bother my doctor. Maybe it was normal? Maybe everyone else was hiding the fact that they had continual tummy ache and felt bloated all the time? And it's not really the kind of thing you want to talk to your friends about. When I did, eventually, go to my doctor, I was told to eat more fiber. It just made things worse.

At long last, I found a specialist who taught me how to manage my food, and also stopped me loading up on fiber. By cutting out certain foods, then reintroducing them to my diet one by one, I found out what I really shouldn't be eating. Now, I've got my IBS under control. Sometimes I do eat food that triggers it off again – we're all human! – but at least I only have the occasional episode. It's no longer the bane of my life.

So that's why I wrote this book. I've been through the wringer with IBS, and I don't see why anyone else should need to. Hopefully, this book can help you live your life with a healthy gut rather than an angry one.

I must make a disclaimer here: I'm not a medical professional. I have looked at the research, but I have sometimes struggled getting my head round it. My expertise is simply that I'm someone who has dealt with these issues in my own life, and found it worth my while getting on top of the jargon and trying to understand the science.

Until recently, most doctors weren't really aware of the importance of gut health. To sketch a metaphor, they knew how to fix all the parts of a car engine, but they didn't realize that if they filled up with diesel instead of petrol, it wasn't going to work!

Some areas, particularly the interaction between the gut and the brain and emotions, are still being researched, and the picture is changing all the time as medical researchers find out more. The gut-brain connection works both ways: living a balanced and unstressed life can help your gut function well, while a healthy gut can help positive feelings. However, poor gut health can lead to a vicious spiral of more stress, leading to worse digestion, leading in turn (in some cases) to depression.

Women are particularly prone to IBS and while some of this may be due to hormonal issues, it may also have a lot to do with the way women are socialized in western society. Women worry about body image, and are often anxious about fulfilling the multiple different roles expected of them and about staying in control of their lives. These stresses set up the beginning of a vicious spiral, particularly when a period of poor health or major physical change (childbirth, menopause) affects their gut health.

The research may not explain everything yet, but the research *is* being done: there's a lot of it out there, and I've read a lot of it over the last few years. You may not have my patience! That's why this book is here.

Most of my suggestions are simple to implement and they can't do you any harm. But it's important if you have persistent problems with your digestion you do speak to your physician and if necessary, have tests to exclude the possibility of more serious conditions.

I'm confident, though, that this book can make a difference to your health. If nothing else, it will help you adopt and maintain a healthy lifestyle. If you get bloated, or have digestive issues, it may be able to help you with those.

And there may be other benefits too. You can reduce stress and negative feelings, and improve sleep, by improving your gut health. You'll be less likely to suffer from other illnesses, as your immune system will be in better shape and able to see them off. If there are coughs and colds going round the office, you may manage not to catch one this time!

If you enjoy this book and find it useful, I would be forever grateful if you could take a few moments to leave a glowing review so that others can find the book and it can help them too.

Chapter 1
A CLOSER LOOK INSIDE YOUR GUT

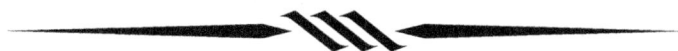

I s it *that* kind of a day? You know, you just had time to snatch a coffee and a croissant for breakfast, you had a meeting that went on for so long that you ended up grabbing a sandwich at three in the afternoon, and you were so tired out when you got home, you just microwaved a lasagne? Or is it the kind of day when you're traveling, and you know you should be eating something healthier, but it was a straight choice at the airport between Burger King and McD's?

Most of us have days like that. Women who have childcare as well as jobs to worry about experience them perhaps more than most! Not only is life stressful, but we're so busy that our best intentions about our diet don't help us. We have to eat *something*, so we end up eating *anything*.

And because you end up with an unbalanced diet, that ends up messing up the bacteria that live inside your intestines – and then that starts to make you sick. It (probably) won't kill you, but it can lead to your feeling bloated all the time, having digestive problems, or just feeling below par, tired, and worn out.

So how does that work? Let's take a look at how your digestive system operates, and you'll soon see why being stressed and eating badly can create a vicious spiral of just getting more stressed and feeling worse about it.

Your digestive system works within your gastrointestinal (GI) tract, which goes all the way from your mouth to your anus. It includes your esophagus, which is where you swallow, and delivers food from your mouth to your stomach; then comes your stomach, the small and large intestines, and anus. We can also break down the intestines into different parts:

- The small intestine is made up of the duodenum, jejunum, and ileum, in that order.

- The large intestine includes the appendix, cecum, colon, and rectum.

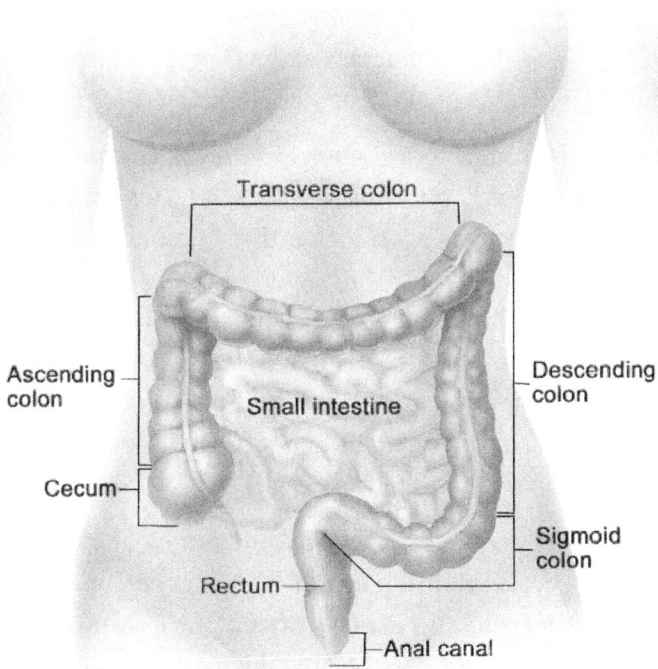

The small intestine is coiled up in the middle of your abdomen. That's where your food is digested and nutrients enter your bloodstream. Then the large intestine makes a sort of cup shape around the small intestine, going up (the ascending colon), across the top (the transverse colon), and down (the descending colon). This is where food that hasn't been digested and absorbed into the body as nutrients ends up, and the waste matter is passed down into the rectum until you feel the need to... er... deal with it, at which point the anus needs to do its job.

The appendix is an odd thing. It's a finger-shaped little pouch attached to the cecum, and we don't actually know what it does. *Probably* nothing, which is why if there is any danger at all of the appendix being troublesome, medics tend to get rid of it first and ask questions later (a burst appendix can be life-threatening – I know, I almost had to have mine removed as a child!).

Although most of the work of digestion happens in the GI tract, other organs are involved in the process too, including the liver, pancreas, and gallbladder. They work together to assist the GI tract in breaking down your food into nutrition in a form your body can use.

The food is moved through your system in a process called 'peristalsis'. This is like continually squeezing toothpaste in a very long tube: the muscles of your GI tract squeeze the food forward a little bit at a time. After food passes through the esophagus, the lower esophagal sphincter closes to stop anything coming back. Then the stomach mixes up the food with digestive juices. This mixture (called chyme) travels into the small intestine, which is helped by the pancreas and liver. The nutrients, digested in the form of sugars, glycerol, amino acids and fatty acids, pass through the wall of the small intestine into your bloodstream.

Imagine the waving tentacles of a sea anemone, or thousands of tiny wiggling fingers. This is what the inside of your small intestine looks like: millions of *villi* that increase the surface area of the intestinal wall and allow nutrients to enter your blood. All the little wigglers grab on to the nutrients and suck them up.

Once the nutrients have been taken out, the large intestine takes the remaining waste and packages it up neatly ready to be excreted.

This is only the basic level of function of your digestive system, though. It also includes a lot of nerves, which for instance communicate with your salivary glands. When you see or smell food, your mouth waters, and your saliva doesn't just moisten the food so you can swallow; it also contains enzymes that help break the food down.

The enteric nervous system, which is contained within the walls of the GI tract, meanwhile keeps sending signals to control the actions of your gut muscles, as well as telling you "Hey, you should find a bathroom sometime soon."

What I haven't mentioned in this anatomical description, though, is the multitude of microorganisms that occupy your GI tract. It's a bit like talking about an office building as being where work gets done, without mentioning any of the people who actually work there. These microbiota play a huge part in getting your gut's work done.

There aren't so many of them in the stomach, where the digestive acids are pretty strong and not many microbes can survive for long, but the lower down the GI tract you go, the more bacteria you'll find. In the small intestine, they're working really hard.

Although you're probably not conscious of much that's going on, your brain is actually talking to your GI tract all the time via the enteric nervous system (ENS), which has more than 100 million nerve cells lining your GI tract. It's a two-way communication. Your feelings can affect your digestion: 'stomach-churning,' 'gut instinct,' or 'butterflies in your stomach' aren't just figures of speech. And your digestion, if it's not working well, can cause depression or anxiety.

That can become a vicious spiral, and I think that's why I started having IBS when I began working. You're stressed or anxious, so that sends a message to your GI tract, which responds by not working properly, which then sends a signal to your brain that makes you even more stressed...

That becomes a negative feedback loop. Stress can also mean that you experience abdominal pain more severely than someone who's not stressed, and again, this can make a big difference to your mood.

So, good gut health is important. First of all, you don't want to feel bloated, you don't want to feel gas or heartburn, or be constipated, or have sudden attacks of diarrhoea. You don't want to get flatulence, which is socially worrisome even if it's not such a serious health issue (I know, I have been there).

Secondly, you probably want to manage your weight. Here, you should know that the microbiota in your gut decide whether you should feel full or hungry. They do this by deciding the amount of short-chain fatty acids that your gut should produce. If your microbiota are out of balance, you might feel hungry all the time, and that can make you overeat. If you never seem to be able to lose weight, your gut microbiota might be the reason.

If you don't have a healthy gut, you may feel deprived of energy. An interesting experiment found that mice who had no gut microbes were lethargic. They simply couldn't get any energy out of their food, however much they ate. A further experiment transferred gut bacteria from depressed people into lab rats. After a while, the rats began to act as if they were depressed, suggesting that they were no longer able to get all the nutrients they needed.

What you eat can be important. Dr. Kirsten Tillisch, a professor of medicine at the University of California, showed that eating live yogurt (which is full of microorganisms) affected the area of women's brains that is associated with processing emotion. She went on to show how this was linked to specific types of gut bacteria. So again, there appears to be a direct link between your gut and your emotions.

A University of Missouri School of Medicine study showed a strong link between IBS and anxiety or depression. Patients with IBS had double the rate of anxiety and depression found in people without IBS. Another study showed sleeplessness can also result from an out-of-kilter gut.

And it's worth noting that 95% of the body's serotonin is made in the gut – that's the chemical that makes you feel good. In addition, one of your gut microbia, lactobacillus acidophilus, gets gut wall cells to produce cannabinoid and opioid receptors. Let's put that into everyday language: it helps to reduce your *perception* of gut pain.

Even if you feel fine emotionally, inflammation in your gut can lead to inflammation elsewhere in your body. That can be associated with skin conditions such as eczema and psoriasis, dandruff, dry skin or acne. Seventy percent of the immune activity in the body happens in the gut, so good gut heath reduces your chances of catching coughs and colds!

Some studies have also found correlations between gut health and autoimmune diseases, cardiovascular disease, and even cancers. Not all of these are a 100% proven, but there's a lot of research work going on in these areas.

Gut health and women

Women have far more IBS than men. Why is this?

One simple reason is that women have more packed into their abdomens than men do. Your colon has to manage to make its way round the uterus and ovaries, so it's a bit twistier than a male colon. Then childbirth, whether natural or caesarian, can have an impact on your digestive system. Ovarian surgeries, pelvic floor dysfunction, or hysterectomies can all affect your GI tract.

Another reason women are more prone to IBS is that their different hormones affect the way the GI tract works. That's particularly the case when the hormones are changing, such as during pregnancy or menopause, or depending on where you are in your menstrual cycle. For instance, you may be more sensitive to pain from your GI tract around the time of your period. On the other hand, increased production of the hormone progesterone in other phases of the cycle can slow the digestive system down, causing bloating and constipation.

Women are also more sensitive to irritants. For instance, women tend to get worse heartburn than men. That may also make you more sensitive to medications. Until recently, most medication recommendations were based on the idea of a male patient as 'normal,' so a lot of women ended up with more than the ideal dosage. Women also appear to have a stronger gut-brain connection, so again, this makes them more prone to IBS and other GI tract issues.

Understanding hormones

Hormones are message packets on your internal communications network, carrying messages from hormone-producing glands (the endocrine system) to different parts of your body. Hormones manage processes which control your appetite, growth, stress, blood sugar, sleep, libido, and even heart rate. Some of them are neurotransmitters, like serotonin and dopamine; that is, they can control your mood. A testosterone or estrogen imbalance can lead to painful periods or even endometriosis, or can inhibit ovulation.

Estrogen also helps to regulate body fat. This is a good example of how poor gut health can affect other parts of the body. A good gut microbiome should produce a certain level of betaglucuronidase, which helps keep estrogen at the right level. If your gut is out of balance, it will allow estrogen to be absorbed back into the bloodstream, so that there's too much of it available to your body.

A compromised digestive system can also lead to impaired nutrient absorption, as you don't have the right mix of bacteria to be able to break down certain types of food and turn them into inputs for other bodily functions. A nutrient deficiency can cause a hormone imbalance, because your endocrine system lacks the right nutrients to work on, so can't make the right mix of hormones.

Polycystic ovary syndrome (PCOS) affects up to 10% of women, and is a common cause of infertility. It can interfere with your ability to ovulate, make your periods irregular, cause acne or facial hair growth, complicate pregnancy, or lead to chronic inflammation. While there are plenty of theories about what causes PCOS, recent research indicates that poor gut health could be a trigger.

Women who have PCOS generally have a less diverse microbiome, and have higher levels of some 'bad' bacteria, than women who are free of the syndrome. While there's no cure, it can often be controlled through diet and exercise, in particular making sure there's enough fiber in the diet, and perhaps using a good probiotic supplement.

Another reason that women can be particularly at risk of intestinal health problems is that hormonal birth control (e.g., combined pills which contain estrogen and progesterone) can affect the gut biota.

There is profound gender inequality in healthcare. For instance, while women in the European Union live longer than men, they also spend a greater proportion of their lives with health problems. Research on women's health issues is often poorly funded, and most medical studies are either male-only or based on 'gender blind' clinical testing and trials. Women have only participated in clinical trials from the 1980s, so a lot of older research may not be very accurate when it comes to describing female health.

And women often just aren't listened to, particularly when they report pain. There is actual evidence that women's pain is discounted, whereas men are believed when they report pain.

And of course, women nowadays are expected to be superwomen. We're supposed to do it all, being a breadwinner, homemaker, wife, mother, and boss. We're supposed to be good at multitasking, which means no one ever thinks they're piling too much work on you. You may be a trial judge, a top asset manager, or a research scientist, but when you get home, who vacuums the carpet? There's a huge gender gap in who does the housework, which came to the fore during Covid when men and women with children had very different experiences of working from home.

If you're going to be superwoman, you don't want to be coping with IBS at the same time.

Chapter 2
THE IMPORTANCE OF MICROBIOTA

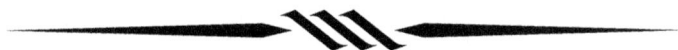

L et's take a closer look at the microbiome and how important it is to your body. There's nothing lovely in what we call our gut. 'Gut' just sounds so horrible; although it's no longer the standard medical usage, I rather like the sound of 'intestinal flora.' It sounds like having a lovely garden growing inside you.

And like all gardens, it needs to be weeded, and it needs to be fertilized, and a lot of this book will be about understanding how to do that.

The gut microbiome plays a major part in keeping you healthy, so let's find out why.

Your gut microbiome includes trillions of microorganisms. Most of these are bacteria. In fact, you are more bacteria than human! (The human body contains an average of forty trillion bacterial cells and only thirty trillion human ones). But the microorganisms in your gut also include fungi of various sorts and even viruses. These help you break down and digest food, and absorb and synthesize nutrients.

In a healthy body, there is a balance of microbiota, mostly symbiotic (living together for the benefit of both organisms, like a good marriage) and some pathogenic (disease-promoting). You may not like the sound of the pathogenic microorganisms, but as long as they are kept in balance with beneficial ones, there is no problem. It's when the balance is disturbed that 'dysbiosis' happens and the normal relationships of these different microbiota can change.

The mixture of all these microbiota is the microbiome, and it's unique to each individual. You won't have quite the same mix as anyone else. In fact, there's a huge diversity of different microbiomes. They're all over your body, on your skin, in your mucous membranes, but the biggest load of microbiota is in your gut.

That's one thing that has made the microbiome quite difficult for scientists to analyze, until recently. Imagine you wanted to establish which species of tree there were in a forest. You could go to the forest, walk around and note down the numbers of each kind of tree you saw. You could even just take a sample; if you expected all the parts of the forest to be similar, you'd only need to catalog one acre, not all 110 acres, and take that as an average. You'd likely only find a dozen kinds of tree anyway, making it a simple job.

But with trillions of microorganisms in the human gut, and over 1,000 different species, sampling isn't easy. These microorganisms encode, altogether, about three million genes; the human genome is much simpler with just 23,000 separate genes. It's only now we have technology such as genetic sequencing machines and computational analysis that we can sample the microbiome. Now we know a lot more about how it works.

For instance, while you were a toddler, you probably tried eating mud, dirt, or grass. Guess what? You will have added some new microbes to your gut. But by the time you grew up, your gut microbiome was likely relatively stable.

The adult microbiome tends not to change much, but there are exceptions to this rule. If you change your diet – like a friend of mine who went to live in Japan, where food is very different – then your gut microbiome can change quite markedly. If you're ill, that can also bring about changes in your gut, particularly if you take antibiotics.

The microbiome develops very early in life; it may even begin in the womb. As I mentioned earlier, many factors influence your microbiome in your early life: genetics, the way you were born (caesarian or natural birth give exposure to different microbes), bottle or breastfeeding. As you grow, stress, diet, periods of illness, drugs (particularly antibiotics), and lifestyle all affect the balance. If you're unlucky, some kinds of good bacteria could be completely killed off.

Now let's look at what your gut microbiome does for you. It can stimulate your immune system, helping your body repel diseases. It synthesizes vitamins and amino acids; in fact, only bacteria can create vitamin B12, as they are the only microorganisms that possess the right enzymes to do it. It can break down complex carbohydrates to form short-chain fatty acids (SCFAs), a nutrient source that helps muscle function.

SCFAs are also important for strengthening the gut barrier function. That's the ability of your GI tract walls to keep your intestinal contents and processes separate from the other things going on inside your body. You really don't want stuff from your gut going straight into the bloodstream before your microbiome has got to grips with it and turned it into nutrients. 'Leaky gut' is a problem for many people, and often happens when highly processed foods, such as artificial sweeteners, destroy beneficial microorganisms and compromise the gut lining. SCFAs also help fight inflammatory diseases – butyrate is a particularly important component here.

Your gut microbiome also specializes in breaking down fiber. That's something that's unique to your gut bacteria; other kinds of microbiota can't do it. And you have various gut microbiota that fight against pathogens, for instance, if you have eaten contaminated food. Each one tends to specialize in fighting off a particular kind of enemy.

You may ask, "What is a healthy microbiome?" It's impossible to specify a particular formula, but for your microbiome to work well you'll need a good diversity of bacteria – up to 1,000 species, each playing a slightly different role. Ideally, you'll want redundancy – that is, two or three different microorganisms that play the same role – so if any of them weaken or die off, there are others to do the job. While each type of bacteria has a job to do, and sometimes two or three, it's the microbiome as a whole that is important. You could compare it to a society: each individual has certain roles, like mother, banker, bus driver, student, but society can't work unless it's got the right mix of roles. If everybody decided to become a student, our public transport system would break down, and the shops would be empty within days.

Heliobacter pylori, for instance, has two effects. One isn't beneficial: it can trigger ulcers. But the other is very useful: it can help regulate your appetite. It lives in a gut microbiome that can predispose the bacteria to doing one job rather than the other, or with other bacteria that will protect your intestinal lining.

Fortunately, it's easier to promote this diversity than to implant any one type of microorganism. It's more like creating a garden than firing a magic bullet!

Sometimes we hide the effects of poor gut health with medicines. Unfortunately, this can actually make things worse rather than better. Some medicines taken for other conditions can also affect your GI tract in various ways.

For instance, non-steroidal anti-inflammatory drugs (NSAIDs) are used for many conditions, including painful periods, sprains, strained muscles, and headaches; they're also used to help treat long term conditions like arthritis that can cause pain. The problem with NSAIDs is that they can irritate the lining of the stomach, weakening its ability to resist stomach acids and leading to inflammation (gastritis), ulcers, bleeding, or perforation of the stomach lining. These conditions can be serious – much more serious than the original reason for taking the NSAID! – so if you need to take NSAIDs and you have a history of ulcers or gastritis, make sure your doctor knows about it.

Other drugs may slow down your digestion or even cause constipation (that's why patients hospitalized after surgery are often given Movicol or a similar laxative). Drinking plenty of fluids and increasing the proportion of fiber, whole grains, fresh fruit and vegetables in your diet can help with this issue.

Antibiotics, on the other hand, can cause diarrhoea. This is because they affect the composition of the microbiome, allowing the Clostridium difficile (C.difficile) bacteria to become prevalent. C.difficile is always there, but it should be only a small part of the total microbiome. If it grows too fast, it can cause colitis, an inflammation of the intestine that causes diarrhoea. If you do take antibiotics, ensure you also have a probiotic such as kefir to ensure good microbiome.

These relationships between different medications and the gut microbiome aren't always at the top of a medical practitioner's mind. In fact, a lot of the research on the subject is relatively recent, so if your doctor is neither young nor an avid reader of new research, they may have missed out on it. It's up to you, then, to ensure that if your doctor is prescribing you medication for another condition, you bring up the issue of the effect on your digestive system.

THE MICROBIOME AND YOUR LIVER

The human liver and stomach are connected and have a significant relationship. The GI tract sends digestive products called *metabolites* to the liver, and the liver sends bile (digestive acid) back to the stomach. So this should be a circular system, but it can be knocked out of whack by dysbiosis.

Let's take a look at how that works. Some bacteria make inflammatory metabolites. When your gut microbiome is healthy, they're in a small minority; when it's not, they're more prevalent, and if the intestinal barrier has also been weakened ('leaky gut'), it will probably let more of these problem bacteria and their metabolites into the portal vein that leads to the liver. That can lead to a damaging immune response, and can be a trigger for non-alcoholic fatty liver disease (NAFLD). Twenty-five percent of Americans have non-alcoholic fatty liver disease (NAFLD), so it's a big problem.

In 2020, probiotics which help stimulate the gut flora were endorsed by Espen (the European Society for Parenteral and Enteral Nutrition) as a treatment for fatty liver disease. Both prebiotic and probiotic supplements targeting the gut microbiome are now being studied as ways of helping.

Food for the microbiome

So you can see how important the gut microbiome is for your body. It's essential that you're careful about what goes into your gut; nutrition is one of the most important levers for health, along with exercise. However, to get to where you want to be, you can't just follow a list of top ten foods to avoid, or add a particular supplement, or decide to eat superfoods like goji berries. There is no magic bullet!

We can say, though, that evidence shows that eating a Mediterranean style diet, with plenty of fruits, nuts and vegetables, and relatively low amounts of dairy product, is good for gut health in general. A Japanese or Korean-style diet, with plenty of fermented foods such as miso, kimchi and pickles, can also stimulate a healthy gut. Important characteristics of healthy eating also include:

- Low sugar intake.
- High fiber.
- Plenty off unsaturated fats such as olive oil, peanut oil, avocados, nut and seed oils.

These are the foods that beneficial bacteria like to eat, so you are encouraging the right bacteria within your microbiome.

There are a few myths around, too, about what you need to eat to have a healthy digestive system. Let's take a few of those to task.

MYTHS

- "You can't eat cheese, you can't drink coffee, you need to cut out gluten..." While some people do have intolerances (lactose being a common one), getting good health is about eating the *right balance* of food, not cutting out food groups.

- "A food intolerance test will tell you what you need to do to get your gut healthy." Apart from the fact that most of these tests are scientifically disputed, look again at that first point. Cutting things out is not *automatically* going to help.

- "You need a colon cleansing/colonic irrigation." Actually, this could get rid of quite a lot of your 'good' bacteria, so it's a lousy idea. As for 'detoxing,' that's what your liver and kidneys and your 'good' bacteria are all supposed to be doing for you.

There is no standard plan for a gut-healthy diet. In fact, there's an increasing amount of evidence that you'll need to make a personalized plan, because no one has exactly the same gut microbiome or exactly the same needs. You have a unique bacterial footprint, just like you have unique fingerprints (Scientific American says the chance of two people having identical fingerprints is 1 in 64 trillion!). You also have unique genes. So a personalized nutrition plan looks sensible.

This is an area where some ground-breaking research is now being carried out, along with genomics (the study of the individual's genetic makeup) and proteomics (the study of proteins within your body, how they're created and how they interact). Another growth area of research is metabolomics – the study of metabolites, outputs of the digestive process which exist as small molecules within cells or organisms.

Elite athletes have been using personalized diet plans for a while. Diet interventions are based on data analyzing what they eat and how they respond to it. Now, similar approaches are becoming more widespread for those of us who run our marathons over the five hour mark, or don't run marathons at all, or even run for the bus!

Our genetic makeup affects how and what we eat and how our bodies respond to it. For instance, some people can metabolize caffeine easily, others can't. Cutting out caffeine can therefore transform some people's lives, while other people might not notice any difference. So if you find what works for you, it may not be exactly the same as what works for your best friend or even your siblings.

Some companies are already offering microbiome data sourced from stool tests or blood tests as a basis for personalized advice. That's certainly in line with what the research suggests. However, it's not obvious how all the tech works, and some companies are using the tests to provide only the kind of good advice you could get from a book on nutrition, or to sell their own supplements. Only a few such companies have scientific back-up in the form of research papers. Be cautious if you decide to use such a service, and check out the scientific validation before you try it out.

Record your symptoms

But the idea of treating yourself as a scientific experiment is not a bad one. Let's adopt the scientific method in terms of trying to solve your gut health issues. That means first defining the problem, then trying various solutions and seeing what works.

First of all, know your symptoms – both objective signs (such as diarrhoea) and subjective symptoms (such as generally feeling low). Objective signs such as high blood pressure or a heart murmur can be detected by investigation; subjective symptoms are things only you know about, such as mood, aches and pains.

Now think about whether those symptoms are intermittent (relapsing from time to time) or whether they are chronic (long-term, stable conditions). Write down what the issues are. Note your feelings, if you are stressed, anxious, or feeling low. Note any pain or cramp in your abdomen, any feeling of bloatedness or gassiness. You might want to note how such symptoms relate to your menstrual cycle.

Start a food diary

That's the first stage of record keeping. Now let's move on to the second: start keeping a food diary. There's no need to be judgmental here. You are simply going to make a list of what you're eating and drinking, and how much of it. You need to be really specific. For instance, don't just put 'chicken,' but note whether you had fried chicken in batter, poached chicken with cream sauce, chicken nuggets, or steamed, skinless chicken breast. Note down extras such as sauces, dressings, and how much sugar you put in your tea.

It can be useful to note when you ate, where, and in what company – with family, with friends, or late in a hotel bedroom with a room service club sandwich. You may find that if you're traveling for work, you don't always have the healthiest eating habits when you're away; maybe having found that out, you can think about how to solve the problem. Also, note down your mood when you ate ('excited,' 'feeling down,' 'okay,' 'tired'). Your mood can have an impact on how much you eat or drink, particularly if you're just snacking because you're bored, or heading for a sugar hit because you're feeling tired at work.

Fill in your food diary *when you eat,* not later. That way it will be more accurate!

Keep referring back to your food diary, as it's a really good resource. For instance, if it shows that particular foods always seem to be followed by bloatedness or other digestive issues, try leaving them out for a while and see if it makes a difference. It can also be useful to show a doctor if you have issues.

Think about what you're eating. Do you get enough diversity in your diet? This can be difficult, especially if you're vegetarian or vegan, or have other food restrictions to follow. Do you get enough fruit, veg, pulses and whole grains? That can be difficult if you're busy, or have faddy kids... Eating the same few things all the time is not great for your microbiome. And lack of diversity is a real, global problem: 75% of the world's food supply comes from just twelve plants!

If your diet is not very diverse, try some different foods to improve your diet diversity. For instance, try vegetables from a different region, such as Indian gourds, African yams and beans, South American sweet potatoes or quinoa, Korean kimchi and different Chinese greens. If you have potatoes with every meal, try some rice from time to time.

Make sure you get fiber in your diet. Good sources are lentils, chickpeas, beans, and oats, as well as asparagus, Jerusalem artichokes, leeks, and onions. Eat nuts rather than chips as a snack, and try to buy bread and pasta that contains whole grains (e.g., 'brown' bread) instead of processed grains. You might also try to increase the diversity of grains you're eating by buying a multigrain, rye or kamut bread.

There is a whole chapter on dietary supplements later, so I won't talk a lot about it here. However, it's worth mentioning that a study of obese women found that taking a daily prebiotic supplement for three months increased healthy bacteria in the gut and could help with their weight reduction efforts.

SUMMARY – TIPS FOR KEEPING A FOOD DIARY

1. Get to know your symptoms and their frequency.
2. Keep a food diary of what you are eating and drinking.
3. Note when you ate, where, and in what company.
4. Note your mood when you eat.
5. Note any symptoms when you eat certain foods.
6. Think about what you're eating and if your diet is not diverse, try different foods.

The importance of exercise and sleep

Another important factor in helping your gut health is physical activity, although we're not yet sure why. Professional athletes, for instance, have more diverse gut flora than less active people; in fact they have double the number of different families of bacteria, as well as higher levels of the beneficial Akkermansia bacteria, which can help prevent obesity.

Getting good sleep and eating regular meals also helps gut health as well as helping your health generally. Your body tries hard to establish a regular circadian rhythm (twenty-four-hour cycle), and it doesn't like that rhythm to be disturbed. There are some indications, too, that sleep deprivation can mess up your microbiome.

I know that this is a big ask if your lifestyle isn't already a super-healthy one. Changing habits can be hard. It can be particularly difficult if you don't have any system in place to help. But it's actually harder to stop a bad habit than it is to create new good ones.

Partly, that's because if you have a bad habit, you feel you're being accused of having no willpower, being unable to help yourself, and so on. Our society can be terribly judgmental, which is why we have such problems helping people with mental health issues. Shame and stigma don't help motivate you to change.

We will talk more about exercise and sleep later in the book.

Changing habits

So let's take a different approach to habit-changing, using a basic psychological response. Your brain works this way: if neurons fire at the beginning and end of a behavior, then they will eventually make it into a habit. So that means your habits are engraved in your memory. Having automatic habits is helpful – for instance, not having to think about "how am I walking? Which foot should I move now?" or "Okay, I'm getting up; now I need to go brush my teeth."

The bad news is that your bad habits have been hard-wired that way. The good news is that you can also create new habits, and once you've got them going, they will be hardwired too. Use incentives to start those new habits. Hold yourself to some basic accountability, and your life will start to change for the better as those new habits get easier and easier to maintain. There is some research to show that habits can be formed in just twenty-one days.

You now know just how important the gut microbiome is, particularly to women, and you may already have a good idea of the habits you might need to change in order to get your gut good and healthy.

In the next chapter, we'll look at some of the signs of poor gut health, and their causes and effects, in more detail.

ACTION STEPS

1. Keep a record of any symptoms that might indicate your gut health isn't as good as it could be.

2. Start a food diary and see what triggers you.

3. Add a new vegetable or fruit to your shopping basket every week.

4. Find a diversity short-cut, such as making your own muesli with different kinds of nuts, grains, and seeds, or trying different cuisines from around the world.

5. If you're not already taking regular exercise, start with a short walk every day.

Chapter 3
THE MOST COMMON GUT PROBLEMS

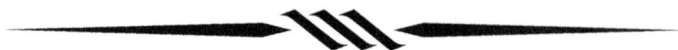

A whole load of things can go wrong with your gut. I don't want to scare you, but you ought to be aware of the commonest GI issues, so you know what's happening if things do go wrong.

Gastrointestinal diseases can be divided into two types: functional and structural.

Functional

Functional disorders are those where the gut is not working properly, but there is no actual change in the organs or tissues of the body. The gut looks completely fine; it just isn't working properly. Functional gut disorders are characterized by chronic gastrointestinal signs and symptoms such as abdominal pain, diarrhoea, constipation, bloating, indigestion, and difficulties with swallowing. Testing would not reveal that your bowel is obstructed or that you have an ulcer. Rather, functional diseases appear to stem from a problem in the gut–brain interaction, causing sensitivity in the GI tract.

Uncoordinated spasms of your gut muscles can cause a range of symptoms from nausea and abdominal pain to vomiting and diarrhoea; or you may simply have increased sensitivity to gastric pain (visceral hypersensitivity). Alterations in your gut microbiome might change your gut's ability to filter out harmful microorganisms and pathogens, while changes in the gut-brain relationship due to stress or depression could affect the time it takes for your digestive system to work.

Common causes include family history, gut sensitivity, a slowing down or speeding up of your gastrointestinal system, a compromised immune system, anxiety, depression, and stress. Generally, medical professionals will try to start by treating the problem with diet and lifestyle changes. Then, depending on the severity of the problem, various medications may be prescribed, and psychological approaches are also sometimes used to get at the root of the problem.

IBS is one of the commonest of the functional disorders. It can include symptoms such as bloating, cramping, and changed bowel patterns; you might experience only one of the symptoms, or a number of them. Often, it's started by dysbiosis, when the gut bacteria get out of balance, or by low-grade inflammation (which might, for instance, have started with an episode of food poisoning). It may also start with changes in the immune response, or medications which change your gut microbiome. It can also lie low for a while, then flare up, triggered by stress, or by eating a particular food.

IBS affects women more than men; estrogen therapy (for instance, at menopause) is also a risk factor for IBS. And intriguingly, IBS is a bigger problem for younger people: those under fifty are far more likely to have it. But while IBS can make your life uncomfortable, like functional disorders, it's not life-threatening.

However, many functional disorders have similar symptoms to structural disorders. So even if you think you have IBS, it is worth talking to a doctor, who may decide to run a number of tests to ensure you don't have a more serious disease. Imaging tests such as ultrasound can find whether you have cancer or an obstruction, for instance; blood tests can also detect serious illnesses.

Structural

Structural disorders are those where tests show that your GI tract is abnormal. For instance, you may have a bowel obstruction, where for some reason your bowel's course is interrupted and it can't continue past a particular point. That will need to be resolved surgically. Other structural disorders include colon polyps, colon cancer, inflammatory bowel disease (IBD), stenosis, hemorrhoids, ulcerative colitis, fistulas (often the result of earlier surgery), and Crohn's disease.

Treatment of structural disorders often involves surgical removal. Not all structural disorders are serious. Hemorrhoids (dilated veins around the anus) can often be made much less painful just by using hydrocortisone cream, and eradicated by healthy bowel habits (e.g., don't strain too hard) and proper diet. While they can make visiting the bathroom a painful experience, they are not likely to kill you. More serious hemorrhoids can be tied off using a ligature, or surgically removed – but the latter is needed in only a small minority of cases.

However, there are some fairly serious diseases included in the list, which is why medical checks are recommended, particularly if you have symptoms such as blood in your stool, constant tiredness, or unexpected weight loss. Screening is particularly useful, since many more serious diseases can be avoided completely if early action is taken. For example, almost all colorectal cancers begin as benign polyps. If screening shows you have polyps, they can almost always be removed painlessly, which is likely to prevent cancer ever developing.

LEAKY GUT

Leaky gut, or intestinal permeability, is still a hypothetical condition – some medics regard it as a disease in itself, while others are less sure. In many cases, it's seen as a symptom of another disease.

Your gut is semi-permeable, rather like a coffee filter, letting some things (nutrients and water) through into your bloodstream while retaining other things (bacteria, fiber, etc.). However, some people appear to have gut walls that have become more permeable, and let through larger particles too, which may be toxic. If the intestinal wall is no longer acting as an efficient barrier, it's putting your immune system in peril.

While leaky gut isn't a recognized diagnosis or a disease in itself, excessive intestinal permeability is a recognized feature of a number of autoimmune diseases such as IBD and celiac disease. It can also cause chronic inflammation of the intestines. It's usually thought to be a symptom, not a cause: because these diseases cause inflammation, they gradually erode the intestinal walls. But some researchers think it may also contribute to triggering some of these diseases.

While research has shown that leaky gut is often associated with these diseases, and may well be an early sign of them, it has not demonstrated that it causes them. Leaky gut can also be caused by chemotherapy, overuse of NSAIDs, chronic inflammation, or some food allergies.

If your gut microbiome is out of balance or under attack, you can get peptic ulcers, or SIBO (small intestinal bacterial overgrowth) which gives you gas and diarrhoea. Your digestion will suffer and you may experience pain in your gut.

The only way to treat leaky gut is to remove the root causes. If it's caused by an underlying condition, such as celiac disease, then your doctor will want to treat the disease, not the leaky gut. The same courses of action advised later in this book to help maintain a healthy gut, such as probiotic and prebiotic supplements, and reducing sugar intake, will also help with intestinal permeability.

Ulcerative colitis

Ulcerative colitis causes irritation and ulcers in your large intestine. It's a form of inflammatory bowel disease, which usually starts in the rectum (as ulcerative proctitis). It then spreads to the large intestine. Its severity and exact location varies from person to person; half those who experience it will only have mild symptoms from time to time. Others, however, will experience bloody diarrhoea and painful abdominal cramps, as well as severe nausea. Sometimes, the disease causes intermittent flare-ups, with no symptoms experienced during the periods between them.

Diagnosis may involve blood tests, stool samples, imaging, and endoscopic tests (sending a small camera up your rectum and colon to take a look). The disease can be treated with corticosteroids, immunosuppressants, or aminosalicylates, but these are generally orientated towards relieving the symptoms rather than eradicating the disease.

Celiac disease

Celiac disease is caused by an adverse reaction to gluten. When a sufferer eats gluten, their immune system will start to attack their own tissues. This damages their small intestine, preventing their body from taking in nutrients properly. It can cause a range of symptoms, including bloating, diarrhoea, and abdominal pain. It can also lead to sudden weight loss, tiredness, and even nerve damage and infertility. Children with celiac disease may have growth problems and even delayed puberty.

Celiac disease tends to affect women more often than men, and can develop at any age. Those with type 1 diabetes, Down's syndrome and Turner syndrome have increased risk of celiac disease, as do relatives of people with the disease. Because its symptoms are similar to those of other diseases, such as IBS, it is often not detected for some time.

Celiac disease is incurable. However, by following a gluten-free diet, celiacs can manage the disease. If the disease is not managed, it can potentially lead to weakening bones from osteoporosis and anaemia, and less commonly, to bowel cancer.

Crohn's disease

This is an inflammatory bowel disease and a chronic condition. Symptoms usually start in early life, and include diarrhoea, cramps, fatigue, weight loss, and bloody stools. Flare-ups can be unpredictable. There is no cure for Crohn's disease, but treatment can mitigate the symptoms of the sickness.

Medications generally include anti-inflammatories such as steroids, and immunosuppressants. Biotherapies similar to those used against rheumatoid arthritis may also be used. These are therapies that use substances from living organisms to treat diseases, with substances that are either naturally occurring in the body or made in the lab. With Crohn's, biotherapies are a class of drugs to manage or treat the disease with biologic or biosimilar medications. Examples of biologics are vaccines, insulin and monoclonal antibodies, all made from living cells. Occasionally, the removal of a small part of the digestive system is proposed.

Crohn's disease may be genetic, since having family members with the disease is a major risk factor. It may also be linked to issues in the immune system in general.

Constipation

Constipation is usually an intermittent problem, but sometimes it can be a longer-term issue. We all have different digestive rhythms, and that includes how often bowel movements occur; however, recurrent constipation can become a serious problem, particularly if your stools become dry and hard, making your bowel movements painful. Fortunately, constipation is unlikely to cause any more serious problems than discomfort.

It's a very common complaint. Pregnant women often suffer from constipation, as the uterus pushes against the colon and slows the passage of waste. Older people may also find their digestive system slows down; if waste doesn't pass through the large intestine fast enough, it may lose so much water that it hardens, making it difficult to pass. Some medications can cause constipation. Eating a diet that is not rich enough in fiber may also lead to problems. It can even arise as a response to a simple change in your regular routine or diet.

Moderate constipation can be managed by self-care. Simple things that can help include drinking more water (and less caffeine and alcohol) and adding more fiber to your diet through eating more fruit, vegetables and high-fiber foods such as bran and oats. Above all, move your bowels when you feel the need to do so; don't try to 'hold it in.'

Anyway, if you read through the whole of this book and put all the advice contained in it into action, you should hopefully avoid constipation for the rest of your life.

Bloating

This is a much less serious issue, health-wise, though it can have a serious impact on your lifestyle and feelings of well-being. Feeling bloated usually reflects the fact that you have a lot of gas in your gut. Most often, this has one of two causes:

1. Food and drink choices that create gas include soda, lots of beans, cabbage soup, fried onions.
2. Swallowing air when you eat, because you eat too fast, or chewing food with your mouth open.

However, bloating could also reflect a digestive problem such as IBS, a food intolerance, or celiac disease. You may also feel bloated around your period.

There are fortunately quite a few things you can do to manage the problem. For instance, you might find massaging your tummy from right to left can help you release trapped wind (from right to left, because that's the direction your digestion goes). Drinking plenty of water can also help, as well as eating more fiber. Try eating smaller, more frequent meals, and see if that reduces the feeling of bloating. Cut out gas-creating foods from your diet.

If you've felt bloated for a whole month, and none of these actions help in reducing the bloated feeling, it's time to see a doctor.

Diarrhoea

Diarrhoea is usually short-lived, and is often caused by eating tainted food or by water-carried infections such as ghiardia. It can also be caused by some medications. However, if it lasts for more than a few days, it usually indicates another problem, such as IBS, or a more serious illness such as Crohn's disease.

For sudden diarrhoea, the most important thing is to ensure you don't become dehydrated, as you are passing a lot of water in your stool. Drink plenty of water. Eating bananas can also help, adding fiber and giving you some basic nutrition. Rice, toast (better than bread in this case) and apple sauce or compote are other foods that can help. Avoid coffee, juice and alcohol, as well as fatty or fried foods.

You may want to take a medication such as Imodium (ioperamide) or Pepto-Bismol (bismuth subsalicylate), which can help stop the diarrhoea. However, don't do this on a long-term basis. In fact, it can be better to let the diarrhoea run its course, since that's the body's way of dealing with toxins, but daily life means that's not always easy to do.

See a doctor if the diarrhoea persists more than three days, or if it is accompanied by a high fever. Also see a doctor if you are in severe pain or if you see blood in your stools.

This chapter has summed up the various gut conditions you might encounter. You have probably realized by now that many of them share the same symptoms. It's very likely, though, that these symptoms are just part of poor gut health.

In the next chapter, we'll look at other signs of poor gut health, which aren't connected directly with your digestive system.

ACTION POINTS

1. It's worth carrying out a little family history research or asking family members if there are any conditions in the family to which you might be genetically predisposed, such as colorectal cancer, celiac or Crohn's disease.

2. Sit down for a minute and think about times you have had poor digestion or other symptoms of intestinal disease. Has it made a big impact on your life? How often have you been really ill as a result?

3. Then make a note of how often you have been in hospital or very seriously ill, and had extensive medication. Can you remember what that did to your digestive system? Did you have stomach upsets afterwards?

4. Work out how much fiber you're getting in your diet right now. How could you improve that? Could you eat one more portion of fruit every day, for instance? Could you switch to brown bread instead of white? To work out how much fiber you're getting now, use an app such as 'MyFitnessPal' to track what you're eating in each day and it will give you the macros.

5. Get ready to read Chapter 4!

Chapter 4
SIGNS, CAUSES AND EFFECTS
OF POOR GUT HEALTH

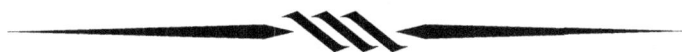

T he Ancient Greek doctor Hippocrates thought that all diseases begin in the gut!

He didn't know everything, but he was the first physician to write down what he knew, and he was quite smart and observant. So while he overstated the case a bit, a lot of chronic diseases *do* actually start off there.

If your intestinal lining is in poor shape, endotoxins – molecules in bacteria you really don't want – can leak through the lining and get into your bloodstream (they are quite nasty things: an acute infection can cause fever or septic shock). Then your immune system goes on the attack, resulting in chronic inflammation. These toxins probably won't leak through in enough quantity to cause infection, but they will eventually stimulate chronic inflammation.

Some have suggested that this inflammation, if it gets worse, can trigger insulin resistance, causing diabetes, and we've already seen how it's linked to fatty liver disease. Plenty of other diseases are also being linked to it, though right now the science is still evolving.

When you have inflammation because a mosquito bit you or you twisted your ankle, and your immune system has responded, that's good – your body is helping you. Inflammation helps to start the healing process. But when the inflammation is caused by your own microbiome, that's counterproductive. It's a bit like hitting yourself and getting bruised – not really a sensible behavior!

Signs of poor gut health

So what does poor gut health look and feel like? Let's explore a few of the signs.

SIGNS OF POOR GUT HEALTH

- Unexplained weight gain or loss, or inability to lose weight however hard you try.
- Unexplained fatigue, even though you're getting the right amount of sleep.
- Insomnia or regular waking throughout the night.
- Skin rashes or acne.
- Sugar cravings; always feeling hungry, even when you've eaten.
- Autoimmune diseases such as rheumatoid arthritis, thyroid issues or type 1 diabetes.
- Depression or anxiety, low libido.
- Heartburn.
- Bloating.
- IBS.
- A sudden change in bowel habits.
- Constipation or diarrhoea on a regular basis.

Note that not all of these symptoms appear to have anything directly to do with your digestive system, but they can still be symptoms of an unhealthy GI tract.

There could also be more subtle signs that you might have poor gut health:

- You're irritable.

- You get headaches, and they're associated with abdominal pain.

- You have bad breath despite regular brushing and good dental care.

- You suddenly have a new food sensitivity that wasn't there before.

If you suddenly have really bad diarrhoea and stomach cramps, it's quite possible you've eaten something bad. You may well be able to identify it. But if you have low-level digestive problems all the time, it's more likely a sign of poor gut health.

Low energy is often a sign of an unhealthy GI tract. Often, a less diverse gut microbiome is found in patients who report overwhelming fatigue. But it takes a bit of detective work to find out why.

An infection or high stress levels can unbalance your gut bacteria, giving pathogenic bacteria like E.coli, enterococcus or streptococcus a chance to cause trouble. These can then start to erode the stomach lining. Continued inflammation eventually deteriorates the lining, letting even more microbial byproducts through. Those in turn stimulate further inflammation and further erosion of the wall, so the problem just keeps getting worse. It's a vicious cycle.

The molecules called cytokines that promote inflammation can start to circulate in the blood and cause problems all over the body. Inflammation stresses the body, which is making an effort to fight off an infection that doesn't actually exist. *That* is the reason you start to feel tired.

Cytokines can also have an effect on the hypothalamic–pituitary–adrenal (HPA) axis. This axis links the three glands that have a big effect on your mood and level of stress. These glands coordinate to release cortisol, which regulates your circadian rhythm. If you don't get enough cortisol, you're going to feel like you haven't really woken up.

Lack of sleep can also be a sign of poor gut health. The composition of your microbiome plays a key part in your stress levels, your mood, and even pain perception, hormones and neurotransmitters. That means your gut could make it difficult for you to get to sleep, or give you low quality of sleep, for instance waking you up with aches and pains.

Causes of poor gut health and an introduction to improving gut health

Diet

A poor diet can be a cause of poor gut health. What can you do about this? Eat better, and get those gut bacteria working!

If you garden, you might have a compost heap, and if you do, you know that it needs a good mix of ingredients to work. You can't just fill it up with grass clippings and expect it to do its job. It needs some brown stuff like paper or twigs, and some green stuff like grass clippings and leaves, and if you don't get the mix right, it will likely go slimy and you'll never turn it into proper compost.

Your gut bacteria need a good mix of material to break down, too. So if you're only eating fast food, they can't do much for you.

Most of us know what we ought to be eating, but we don't stick to it for several reasons. One reason is economic: fresh fruit and vegetables can be costly, while supermarket pizza (for instance) is cheap. Another reason is impulse: when you just know that you want a Ben & Jerry's Chocolate Chip Cookie Dough ice cream, nothing else will do. Sometimes, you don't really want to eat french fries and onion rings, but you know your kids will give you no peace if they don't get them, so you order the same; or you're out to dinner with friends and if everyone else orders a starter and a dessert, you don't want to look like a party pooper.

And sometimes you just don't have time to cook, so you break out a microwave meal from the freezer.

Another reason – let's be honest about this – is that food can be addictive, and a lot of the big food manufacturers know this. Sweet, fatty, and salty are the key addictive flavors; they appeal to the cavewoman in us, when we used to have to eat energy-rich foods because we didn't know when the next meal would be coming. That's why we get cravings. About a fifth of people have real problems with an addictive relationship with food.

If you think 'addiction' is too strong a word, think again. The same drug that's used to block opium overdoses, naxolone, can also block sugar cravings.

Highly processed food and strong flavors can also suppress the satiety mechanism, which is why you can binge till you feel sick. Most addictive foods are sugary and fatty – chocolate, cookies, ice cream, sodas, cake. They are 'more-ish,' and if you've ever binged on ice cream, you know how bad it can get. But pizza and french fries also hit the addictive list.

Oddly, strawberries don't make it to addiction status, even though they are really tasty. Nor do apples or bananas. There is no fat or processed sugar involved, that's why.

Watch out for processed foods such as microwave meals, even if they look healthy. They often contain a high loading of sugar and salt to make them more flavorsome (and addictive). They may also contain additives such as emulsifiers, which can have a bad effect on your gut, and sweeteners such as aspartame, sucralose, and saccharin, which will impact your gut microbiome. Read the printed label and you'll find out what is going on.

Beware of food that appears natural but actually has a high sugar or salt content. Some kinds of dried fruit have lots of added sugar, while roast peanuts are almost always excessively salted, and honey roast cashews present the worst of both worlds. Mueslis, granolas, and trail mixes can also be a lot less healthy than they look.

Sugary food has a really bad effect on the gut microbiome. Sucrose and fructose both block the production of a protein that some beneficial bacteria (specifically, bacteroides, thetaiotaomicron) need. High sugar levels can also affect the microbiome's ability to regulate blood sugar, and in the most extreme cases, this can lead to diabetes.

If you have a restricted diet, such as vegan, crudivore, gluten-free, or any weight loss diet which restricts the diversity of food you're eating, that could also change your gut microbiome. You'll need to make a special effort to ensure you're getting a range of foods, which will help you maintain a diverse gut microbiome.

The diversity of your microbiome affects the availability of nutrients, and also affects the richness of communication between the GI tract and other parts of the body.

Let's take one instance where having a more diverse diet can save you problems. Shellfish, milk, eggs and red meat contain a compound called phosphatidylcholine, which bacteria can convert to trimethylamine (TMA). Your body makes trimethylamine-N-oxide (TMNA) out of that, and it's one of the compounds linked to atherosclerosis, whereby your arteries harden and become clogged.

So you could cut out shellfish, milk, eggs, and red meat completely. That would be one way to prevent your arteries hardening. But some kinds of oil, such as olive oil, and some kinds of vinegar, help to inhibit TMA production. So instead of cutting out shellfish and meat, you could just make sure you use plenty of olive oil and balsamic vinegar in your salad.

COMMON FOODS THAT ARE BAD FOR THE GUT

- Processed sugar (sucrose and fructose).
- Foods high in salt.
- Processed foods.
- Additives e.g., emulsifiers, such as Polysorbate 80, found in sauces and salad dressings, and carboxymethylcellulose or CMC, used as a thickening agent in cheeses, dressings, and even fruit juices and

milk.

- Sweeteners such as aspartame, sucralose, and saccharin.

Not having diverse bacteria in the gut

The more diverse the bacteria in your gut, the more likely it is you'll have ones that do the right thing. Basically, your health concerns the whole community of bacteria, not just individual species. Incidentally, the diversity of the microbiome has been found to drop abruptly in patients just before the onset of Type 1 diabetes. The ecology of gut microbiota is individual to each of us. When different people eat the same food, they experience different amounts of blood sugar spike, because they have different enterotypes (styles of gut microbiome).

Let's compare this to learning a language. If you only know "hello," your ability to respond to an interaction in that language is very limited. Add "How are you?," 'It's nice weather today," and you have expanded your possibilities for interaction. It's not about knowing one word – you really need a few hundred, at least, to start being able to have a meaningful conversation. In the same way, your gut needs a whole vocabulary full of different bacteria to be able to interact with the food you're eating and other parts of your body.

And you get diversity of bacteria by eating a diversity of food. Ensuring your diet provides plenty of probiotics will also help you maintain a good, diverse microbiome. Probiotics are substances which encourage the bacteria in your gut to multiply. They are often a combination of beneficial bacteria (such as lactobacillus and bifidobacterium) and yeast (such as saccharomyces boulardii).

These are often contained in fermented foods such as kimchi, sauerkraut, kefir, yogurt, pickles, and kombucha. Buttermilk and sourdough bread, tempeh and miso also contain probiotics. If you learn to make your own pickles – as many Korean and Japanese families do – you can improve your diet dramatically. You might also choose to take dietary supplements such as Yakult or Actimel, or capsules (note that these are not approved by the

FDA and are therefore limited in the claims they can make).

While probiotic supplements can help your gut, more research is definitely needed. The underlying science is good, but we're not sure how effective particular probiotics are for treating digestive conditions. Some probiotics may need special storage, and can get out of date quickly. You may also find that you have a slight reaction for the first few days you use them, such as a tummy upset, gas, or diarrhoea, so it's important to continue for at least a couple of weeks unless you are feeling very unwell.

If you are immuno-compromised, have a critical illness or have had surgery recently, taking probiotic supplements is probably not such a great idea. However, if you have taken antibiotics while you were ill, taking probiotics later on can be a good way to stimulate your gut microbiome and get it back to normal.

Smoking and drinking

Two things you *shouldn't* do if you want a healthy gut are drink a lot of alcohol or smoke. That probably doesn't surprise you much, as these are the two regular suspects that most medics warn you about with regard to all aspects of your health.

Your body doesn't treat alcohol like other nutrients in food; the body prioritizes getting rid of it. But that involves turning it into a toxic chemical, acetaldehyde. That's one reason alcohol is a known co-carcinogen: it may not cause cancer, but it can facilitate tumors taking hold.

It can also affect stomach acid production negatively, and that can allow harmful bacteria to survive in what you eat and get through to your small intestine. Alcohol can also damage the stomach wall.

Smoking, meanwhile, can weaken the esophagal sphincter, leading to acid reflux or heartburn. And though with don't know exactly why, Crohn's disease is more common in smokers than in non-smokers, and smoking can make it harder to control the disease and its symptoms.

Stress and the gut microbiome

You've probably heard people say "My job is so stressful, I'll end up getting ulcers." Stress can, in the short term, lead to stomach upsets or difficulty swallowing and digesting your food. But it also has longer-term effects on gut health, particularly if it's linked to poor dietary habits. Anxiety can lead to diarrhoea or gas, and stress can trigger intestinal cramps, when your brain sends stress signals to the enteric nervous system (the nervous system which controls your gut).

Short-term stress is one thing, but if you have chronic anxiety, that can make things worse. You can get into a vicious circle: stress makes your digestion worse, and that makes you feel more stressed. No wonder 60% of people living with anxiety or depression have IBS (that's a correlation, not necessarily a cause, though).

A few quick fixes for stress are deep breathing, yoga, stretches, meditation, walking, and self-compassion, but something that can work particularly well is just to ask friends and family to help remind you that you have support from others. We will learn a lot more about dealing with stress, and having a healthier lifestyle, in Chapter 9.

Poor sleep patterns

Poor sleep can lead to gut problems, particularly if you have late nights and irregular bedtimes. If you eat just before bed, you're making things worse: your gut won't get a rest, as it will be trying to digest while you sleep.

Sleep deprivation can also lead to food cravings, in particular a craving for sugar and trans fats, which won't do your digestive system any good. And of course, if you're frustrated by sleeplessness, your stress levels are going to increase, which can also make your gut feel poorly. We'll talk in more detail about sleep in Chapter 10.

How do you know if you have a problem?

There are a number of ways you can scope out a possible gut issue. Some companies now offer microbiome testing. You can get DIY testing packs which can check out your gut microbiome via a stool sample. You send the sample off to a lab for analysis, and your results should be with you in a few days or weeks, depending on the company (and possibly the price). Your results should show what kinds of microbes were found in the sample, along with possible food sensitivities. It can also tell you if inflammatory markers have been found – that's a really good warning of possible health issues ahead.

It's a first step, not a full diagnosis, but a big plus is that you save yourself the embarrassment of having to talk to your doctor, and it's all handled online. The cost of such tests is usually under $200. The downside is that such tests are not FDA approved, and some companies get very poor reviews.

Make sure you do your due diligence before you book a test. Know what exact bacteria or sensitivities the lab looks for, and whether they have clinical studies backing their methodology. Also check out customer reviews, just as you would for any other purchase.

You can also get a stool test done through your regular doctor. If the test is required for specific medical reasons, your insurance will probably pay for it (or you'll get it on the NHS, if you're British). In this case, you'll be getting a test that is FDA approved, and it's likely you'll also be asked for blood tests at the same time to give an all-round view of your health.

When should you call a doctor?

While for the most part the digestive system issues we're talking about in this book are not life-threatening, even if chronic (long-term), there are a few times that you should definitely call a doctor.

If the pain is really severe, you could have a gastric obstruction. That needs immediate surgery. You might have a tumor, benign or cancerous; in both cases, the earlier the growth is removed, the better the prognosis for your health in future. So, severe pain, rather than grumbling tummy, means a visit to the doctor straight away.

If you have difficulty swallowing, or episodes of choking, you need to see a doctor. This can have several causes, such as chronic acid reflux, neurological illnesses, or problems with the immune system, but needs seeing to properly. I'm not talking about getting a fish bone stuck in your throat or choking on your coffee when a friend tells a bad joke; it's when you regularly choke on food with no apparent reason, or when eating makes you start coughing.

If there is blood in your stool, you should certainly see a doctor. Something is not right, and it is possible that you will need either specific medication or surgery. It could also be something minor like haemorrhoids.

Other times that you really need to go see a medical professional are if you have persistent constipation or diarrhoea, lasting more than a few days, or if you experience a sudden and complete loss of appetite.

Effects of poor gut health

The long-term potential impact of poor gut health

I don't want to turn you into a hypochondriac. So please don't read this part of the chapter and convince yourself that having IBS means you're going to get all the diseases I mention. Nonetheless, it's worth knowing the long-term potential impact of poor gut health, so that you can decide it's worth your while treating your gut well. It may be just the motivation you needed.

For instance, specific bacteria in the gut have been linked to strokes (or cerebrovascular accidents) of a particular kind. A study that took samples of fecal matter from stroke victims and compared them to a control group had interesting results. The presence of fusobacterium and lactobacillus was associated with an increased risk of ischemic stroke (where the arteries near the brain fill up with plaque, limiting blood flow to the brain).

Negativibacillus and lentisphaeria bacteria increased the risk of a more severe stroke; and patients who did not have acidaminococcus bacteria had a better chance of a good recovery after three months.

That suggests that if enough research is done on how to replace beneficial bacteria in the microbiome, stroke victims could have a better chance of recovery. Fecal transplantation is one possible answer. An alternative is that freeze-dried compounds of microorganisms could be administered in capsules, helping to modify the microbiome (this research has not yet been published, but was presented at a 2022 scientific conference by Miquel Lledós of the Sant Pau Research Institute, Barcelona).

I've already spoken about the links between poor gut health and depression, and a major, multi-year study of Finnish participants found that morganella and klebsiella are often found to thrive in people who subsequently experience depression (they are also two bacteria that often cause infections in hospital patients).

Unfortunately, science doesn't yet present a way of laser-targeting those two bacteria. So the best we can do is to ensure that a diverse and healthy gut microbiome keeps them in check by other, healthier bacteria.

Parkinson's disease too might start in the gut, as patients with Parkinson's and other neurodegenerative diseases show differences in their microbiomes from healthy people. Early symptoms can include constipation, which sometimes precedes the full onset of Parkinson's by decades. The exact relationship is still not understood, but is now the target of research at Yale School of Medicine. GI problems may also play a part in Alzheimer's and dementia.

Inflammation is a key contributing factor in Alzheimer's, and it's interesting to find that Alzheimer's patients display a distinctive type of gut microbiome, as well as more inflammation markers in their blood samples. Studies show that rats who had fecal transplants from Alzheimer's patients started to do poorly in memory tests. But again we don't yet know exactly how it works or what we can do to reverse Alzheimer's. It is, however, a very promising direction for research.

This chapter has been quite heavy on theory and information. learned about signs of poor gut health and illness they may be related It's particularly interesting that poor health of the gut microbiome appears to be linked to degenerative diseases in the elderly, suggesting that if you look after your gut right now, your gut will look after you in the long term.

The next chapter will be much more practical. We're going to look at eliminating certain food groups from your diet, in order to isolate any food intolerances you may have. That can be a bit of a pain in the short term, but long term, it's often a highly effective way of finding out the foods that cause flare-ups of IBS, for example.

ACTION STEPS

1. I'd like you to think how many habits you have that are not conducive to good gut health. Smoking, drinking alcohol, eating a lot of fast food might figure, as might life circumstances such as working in a stressful environment. On a scale of one to ten – one being really healthy and ten being really unhealthy – where do you think you are right now? And where would you like to be?

2. Are there particular foods or types of food that you find really addictive? Make a list.

3. Now do a little research. The reasons may be obvious: if you adore Ben & Jerry's ice cream, Reese's Peanut Butter cups, and coffee with three sugars in, well, sugar is your thing. They may be less obvious, in which case, go read the small print on the packet.

4. Think about the triggers for your eating these addictive foods: working late, feeling depressed, going out with friends, your children like them... Once you know what the triggers are, you can start to overcome the addiction factor.

5. Go out and try some of the fermented foods mentioned in this chapter, and find which ones you like. Great! You can add them to your diet for a healthy gut.

Chapter 5
FOOD INTOLERANCES

———————◄▓►———————

had to rescue one of my friends from the diet from hell. She had a blood analysis that told her to cut out all red meat, all beans and pulses, all dairy products, all potatoes, aubergines, and tomatoes, all nuts, all gluten, all kinds of oils, all sugars, and all salt. It didn't leave much that she could eat. She couldn't even drink soy milk (beans) or almond milk (nuts). She was feeling miserable; she couldn't work up an appetite for the few things that she could still eat.

Well of course she was feeling miserable! Her gut microbiome must have been completely out of kilter. Imagine all those poor bacteria starving to death!

So I sat her down and asked what seemed to be the worst thing for her in terms of bloating and gas. Milk, she said. I proposed she tried out a diet with everything allowed except dairy products. She perked up. After a few weeks of that, she was practically back to her previous diet, except for replacing dairy with almond milk, and that seemed to work. She had her appetite back, and I hope her GI tract was feeling happier too.

I tell you this to stress the importance of *balance* in your body. Bear that in mind as you read the chapter, because if you're looking to have a healthy gut, the worst thing you can do is to brutalize it. You need to keep it in balance. That will help you have energy, maintain a healthy weight, keep stocked up with the right vitamins, and provide other health benefits too.

A high-fibre diet with plenty of whole grains and not too many saturated fats can help reduce your risk of developing type 2 diabetes. It can also help keep your heart healthy, as can plenty of fresh fruit and vegetables, and eating a portion of oily fish (salmon, mackerel, trout or tuna) every week.

You'll want calcium in your diet to keep your bones and teeth strong. Dairy products will deliver this, but you can also get it from dark green vegetables like kale, spinach and broccoli, or from calcium-fortified soya products or fruit juices. You'll also want to be able to absorb that calcium properly, which means you need vitamin D. You can create your own vitamin D by getting out in the sun, or if you have dark skin or there just isn't any sun (like Iceland in December, which gets five hours if you're lucky) then take a supplement.

I'm also going to mention that fasting can affect your microbiome. Intermittent fasting – that is, reducing your calorie intake a couple of days a week, or not eating between an early dinner and a late breakfast – can really help, as it gives your digestive system the time to recover between periods of active digestion. That will actually change the balance of bacteria in your GI tract.

You don't want too much salt and sugar. You don't need to cut them out entirely, but you want to get the balance right; eating crisps and cookies all day isn't going to help. If you have a sweet tooth, save up all your sugar for a square of really intense dark chocolate for nibbling. If you enjoy cooking, use soy sauce rather than salt for flavor – it has six times less sodium.

However, even if you've got a good balance of diverse foods in your diet, there may be one or two that you react to badly. Some foods will make you feel energized, while others can make you feel sluggish and bloated. Estimates of how many people suffer from food intolerances vary widely from 2% of people to one in five; you might be one of them. So cutting some foods out of your diet can help keep you healthy.

Elimination diet

The way you can do this is by trying an 'elimination diet.' This allows you to identify any food intolerances, sensitivities or allergies. It's a kind of diagnosis.

The way an elimination diet works is by removing foods from your menu. It starts with foods that are known to cause intolerance quite frequently, which you should now have an idea of from keeping a food diary. Later, you can reintroduce them, one by one, and see whether reintroducing the food causes any reaction. If it doesn't, then you're fine with it. If it does, then exclude it again and see how well you get on.

By the way, don't use an elimination diet if you think you have a really serious food allergy, such as some people have to nuts. If you get rashes or hives, or if your throat swells up and you have difficulty breathing after eating a particular food, talk to your doctor about it. Reintroducing a food you're strongly allergic to could trigger an anaphylactic shock, which can be very dangerous or even fatal.

If you have (or have recovered from) an eating disorder such as anorexia or bulimia, you might also decide not to try out an elimination diet; it probably pushes some psychological buttons you really don't want to push.

Once you've decided to try an elimination diet, you start with the elimination phase, taking out the foods that you think might be causing you a problem. Some food types that are known to cause intolerances quite frequently are dairy products, gluten (e.g., in wheat and bread), seafood, eggs, nuts, citrus, and nightshade vegetables (potatoes, tomatoes, peppers, eggplant). Cut them out for two or three weeks. During this phase, you'll be able to see if your gut health improves. Do you feel less bloated? Are you feeling more awake and energetic? If this phase of the diet works, you'll know it. If not, and you're still not feeling right, then there is something else the matter, and you probably should talk to your physician.

Food groups that you could consider eliminating include the following:

- Citrus fruits – oranges, grapefruit, lemon, lime. Don't forget this includes juice.

- Nightshade vegetables – tomatoes, peppers, eggplant, potatoes, dried paprika or cayenne pepper. Watch out for processed foods which include paprika (while potatoes are off the menu, *sweet* potatoes are fine; they're not related to this family even though they share a name with the potato).

- Nuts and seeds – peanuts, sunflower seeds, walnuts, almonds, and so on. Remember to eliminate oils or milks made with them, as well as the nuts.

- Legumes – beans, lentils, peas, soy. This would include soy sauce and miso.

- Sugars – white and brown sugar, honey, corn syrup, chocolate, agave syrup, molasses, maple syrup. Don't replace the sugar with sweeteners, as these can have a bad effect on your gut health. And cut out sugary sodas.

- Dairy products – milk, cheese, yogurt, butter. Watch out for sauces including milk or butter in processed foods or when eating out. You might want to bring back cheese or yogurt first, then milk (or goat's milk, then cow's milk).

- Gluten – wheat, barley, rye, bread, cakes, cookies, beer, pasta. Watch out for starches and vegetable gum used in processed foods; you might not know they're there, so read the label.

- Coffee and tea.

- Alcohol.

- Spices – including relishes and mustards.

- Fats – hydrogenated oils, mayonnaise, spreads, margarine. This means no fried food for a while; steam, roast or boil your food instead.

- Corn (maize to British readers) – this can be an inflammatory agent, and some people are sensitive to it, so miss out corn, corn oil and corn syrup.

When I tried the elimination diet, I realized my triggers were mainly breakfast cereals, carrots, cabbage, broccoli and chickpeas.

You have to be really careful about reading labels. For instance, maybe you take a protein shake in the morning, mixed up with milk. You're missing out dairy, so you take it with water instead. Watch out! It might well have a whey protein powder included in the ingredients, which would mean you're drinking milk even though you thought you had eliminated it.

The same goes for eggs, which find their way into a lot of things you might not expect to have egg in. For instance, when I look at the labels for lots of prepared salads, they include egg in the crab sticks, in pasta or in the dressing. Sandwiches are often made with mayonnaise instead of butter (and yes, mayonnaise is made with egg yolks).

You should also plan your calorie count and vitamins so that you ensure you replace everything you've taken out adequately. If you take out all your normal protein foods, you'll need to eat something else that's full of protein; if you take out all your usual calcium by eliminating dairy products, you need to find another way to provide it. It's worth sitting down for a while before you start and doing some basic math.

You'll also get more out of the elimination phase if you keep a diary. Use a small notebook, and put on the left hand page what you ate, and on the right hand page how you feel. It's worth recording general emotional mood as well as specific digestive issues like gas or bloating – you may feel more energized or more optimistic, for instance.

You're going to be eating with a lot more care and attention now! It's also worth taking the time to eat more mindfully. Taste your food slowly, experience the texture and the aromas of your food. You may notice that cravings disappear as your gut microbiome is beginning to rebalance.

So you're three weeks in, and hopefully you feel great, and now the second phase starts – the reintroduction phase. Add just one of the foods you eliminated back into your diet. Let's say you start with dairy products. Don't hog a whole load of ice cream! Just put dairy back where it usually goes, for instance by buttering your toast in the morning, putting milk in your coffee or having milk with your cereal. Do this for two or three days, and keep aware of how you feel.

In particular, look for symptoms such as rashes, bloating, stomach pain or cramps, or changes in your bowel habits. You might also find that reintroducing a food gives you headaches, that you feel fatigued, have difficulty sleeping, or even that you have pain in some of your joints. If you have these kinds of symptoms, then congratulations; you have found a culprit. You can now eliminate that food again.

Reintroduce the others, again, one food group at a time for two or three days at a time. There may be more than one food that gives you difficulties, so don't assume that the food you already eliminated was the only one.

The whole process should only take five or six weeks. Investing a few weeks in improving your life for years to come is a no-brainer! Though, admittedly, if you are like me, you will get very impatient around the three week mark. Don't worry; that's normal!

If you can cope with a really restrictive diet, it's best to eliminate as many foods as you can to start with. However, that can make life quite miserable, particularly since, for instance, if you exclude dairy, gluten, legumes and nuts all at the same time, your choice of milk substitutes will be very limited.

But there are things you can eat and drink to make your diet more interesting:

- Include lots of fresh fruit – berries, peaches, apricots, mango, grapes, pineapple, for instance, all taste great.
- Fresh veg, particularly green vegetables and carrots that you can eat raw, plus parsnips, pumpkin and squashes.
- Dried fruit such as sultanas, prunes and dried mango can be good,

though watch out for the sugar content of some dried tropical fruits.

- Use rice instead of potatoes or pasta to accompany your meals. You might want to try sushi rice instead of your regular rice for a different texture. Puffed rice cereals can replace granolas and other cereals that contain gluten.

- Rice milk and coconut milk (unsweetened) can replace dairy.

- Smoothies are a fantastic way to get fruit into your diet.

- Replace nuts and peanut butter by seed butters and oils, as well as snacking on pumpkin seeds or sunflower seeds.

- Seaweeds (try a Japanese or Korean store) can add crunch and flavor to rice and veg, and intense flavor to soups.

- Roast or mashed sweet potato can replace regular potatoes with a meal.

If you don't think you have the guts to take on a full elimination diet (pun intended), you might decide to eliminate just three areas of food – say, dairy, gluten, and nightshade vegetables. You'll still want to spend two or three weeks not eating these foods, but then you'll have a much shorter period of reintroducing each food group.

The advantage of doing things this way is that if you do have an intolerance, these are the three most likely areas. By eliminating them but leaving other foods in, you're not going to find your diet horribly unappetising, like the poor friend I mentioned at the beginning of the chapter. Also, if you already have some food restrictions because, say, you're vegetarian, or vegan, this will ensure you don't skip so many foods that you start having problems getting enough nutrients.

Muslim sisters, please don't plan your elimination diet to clash with Ramadan. That's taking on too much at the same time, and besides, it will spoil your iftar!

If you already have a good feel for things that upset your stomach, you might want to tailor an elimination diet to target particular groups. For instance, you might want to just cut out gluten.

Gluten intolerance

While full-blown celiac disease affects just 1% of the US population, between 20% and 40% of adults with food sensitivities will mention gluten as a culprit. In celiac disease, dietary gluten, a protein that's found in wheat, rye and barley, damages the small intestine, and this causes the body to be unable to absorb food properly. That can lead to diarrhoea, bloating, abdominal pain, and longer-term deficiencies such as anemia, vitamin deficiency, and even osteoporosis (brittle bones).

People who have some gluten intolerance often report bloating or changed bowel habits after eating gluten, while a number also report brain fog or fatigue. However, it seems possible that it's not the gluten so much as another component of wheat, known as fructans or fructo-oligosaccharides, that causes digestive problems. Fructans are not easy for the small intestine to absorb, and have fermentable components which can bloat the stomach.

There is also some evidence that gluten activates production of a substance called zonulin, which can open the tight junctions in the small intestine, allowing larger particles to pass through the intestinal wall. In other words, it becomes a specific type of 'leaky gut.' This only seems to happen in people with either celiac disease or IBS.

So a gluten-free diet isn't automatically recommended. But if you have bad IBS, then it may be something that works for you.

When you are excluding gluten, watch out for products such as malt syrup, beer, soy sauce, teriyaki sauce, malt extract, seitan, and 'rusk' (often found in sausages). These all are likely to contain gluten (though tamari, similar to soy sauce, doesn't).

Cross-contamination is an issue for those with celiac disease or other extreme gluten intolerance. Though oats don't contain gluten, if they're processed in a factory with other grains, they may be contaminated with it. If you have a slight sensitivity, it won't matter, but if you need to follow a 100% gluten free diet for medical reasons, only buy oats that are labeled gluten free. 'No gluten-containing ingredients,' on the other hand, is a bunch of weasel words, because it doesn't guarantee the absence of cross-contamination. If you need to be strictly GF, don't buy products that say this.

FODMAPs

These fructans, together with some other carbohydrates, are referred to as FODMAPs and are often responsible for GI problems in IBS patients (FODMAPs stands for fermentable oligosaccharides, disaccharides, monosaccharides and polyols, which is quite a mouthful). FODMAPs on their own are quite innocuous, but if you already have IBS, they will be particularly difficult to digest.

Some medics recommend a low-FODMAP diet to patients with IBS. Without going through all the science of FODMAP groups, particular foods you might want to cut out include:

- Sugar fructose found in wheat products, onions and garlic.
- Sugar galactose from pulses, beans, and cashew nuts (and pistachios).
- Lactose (in milk and yogurt).
- Sugar alcohols (polyols) found in artificial sweeteners and 'low-sugar' products.
- Apples and pears, mangoes, nectarines, garlic, onion, leek, cauliflower, and mushrooms.

Foods you can happily eat, which contain no FODMAPs, include meat and fish, eggs, tofu, rice, bananas, melons, citrus fruits, pineapple, raspberries, strawberries, aubergines, courgette, asparagus, cucumber, tomato, salad greens, pumpkin or squash, bell peppers, chillies, carrots, chard, cabbage, and spinach – plus seaweed (so sushi makes a super low-FODMAP meal).

If a low-FODMAP diet works well for you, then you might want to start reintroducing some of the foods you've missed out. If you get on okay with them, you can carry on eating them. You're using the same principles as the elimination diet, only with FODMAP as your main emphasis.

However, there is one potential weakness to low-FODMAP diets. By reducing the diversity of foods and potentially reducing dietary fiber, such a diet could reduce the diversity of the gut microbiome and actually make things worse. It might be better to try probiotics first, which can help the gut deal better with FODMAPs.

Reactions to gluten and FODMAPs can also be exacerbated by stress, which is one reason you might have flare-ups from time to time.

Other ways to help stay healthy when you have a gluten intolerance are eating a high-fiber diet, avoiding refined carbs (e.g., white bread, white rice, pastries), and taking a probiotic supplement.

Lactose intolerance

Over 65% of us can't actually process lactose well. You can become lactose intolerant if your small intestine doesn't make enough lactase, a digestive enzyme that helps break down lactose. That can sometimes happen after an injury or infection. If your ancestry includes Native American, Asian or African parentage, you have an even greater likelihood of becoming lactose intolerant.

Medical tests can tell you if you're severely lactose intolerant; for instance, blood samples will be taken when you are fasting, and then during the two hours after you drink a liquid containing lactose. Normally, your blood sugar levels should rise as your body processes the lactose; if they don't rise as expected, that could show you are lactose intolerant.

Many people find they are not intolerant of all lactose products; some dairy products have less effect on their digestive system than others. For instance, hard cheese and yogurt contain less lactose than milk; some people can tolerate goat's or sheep's milk cheese, but not cow's milk cheeses.

Be careful about labels. A friend of mine who is lactose intolerant in quite a big way loves the one dairy product she can eat, goat's and sheep's milk cheese. However, one day she was really sick after eating some feta cheese. Every feta she had ever eaten was 100% sheep's milk, or 70%-30% sheep's and goat's milk. When she rummaged in the bin for the wrapper and looked carefully on the back of it to see what had made her ill, she found the small print: "Feta cheese made from cows' milk."

Watch out also for food labels on processed foods that mention powdered milk, milk solids, or whey.

You can also manage a mild lactose intolerance by having dairy with other foods rather than on its own. For instance, you might enjoy a little yogurt with a fruit compote, or have cheese together with fresh grapes, bread, or perhaps some crunchy salad. You might also try lactose-reduced dairy products, which have lactase added. The lactase helps to break down the lactose (sugars) in the milk ahead of time, so your digestive system will have less work to do.

Alternatively, you could take lactase pills or droplets before you eat regular dairy products. This can prep your digestive system so that when the lactose arrives, you're ready to digest it.

If you cut out dairy products completely from your diet, make sure you are getting enough calcium from other types of food, such as leafy green vegetables, soybeans and tofu, nuts and seeds. You can also get calcium-fortified products such as orange juice. Calcium is particularly important for women, and the older you get, the more important it is for strengthening your bones and teeth to avoid brittle bones.

Fasting

This is a slightly different topic from elimination diets, but it might prove a useful way for you to manage your GI tract's health. It has to be said that the jury is still out on fasting, though there is medical research for some types of fasting being beneficial. Unfortunately the whole concept of fasting and 'detox' seems to have appealed to some very dubious characters, who on occasion are making money out of schemes that seem likely to damage rather than improve your health.

The idea is that intermittent fasting regimens (i.e., fasting for distinct periods of time, not all the time) can provide a period of rest and recuperation for your gut. Humans, after all, evolved when food wasn't available 24/7 from a nearby store, but was sporadically supplied and highly dependent on the success of hunting trips or what could be foraged at the time. So we evolved to have guts that like a rhythm of, say, twelve hours 'on' and twelve hours 'off,' and that need their downtime.

There are two kinds of intermittent fasting:

1. **Time-restricted eating**, for instance not eating between breakfast and your evening meal, or eating an early evening meal (Jains don't eat after sunset, which in India is usually about 6pm) and fasting through to breakfast time. The most common one you may have heard of is 16/8 intermittent fasting, where you eat for eight hours and fast for sixteen hours. This can also be varied so 12/12 or 14/10 for example.

2. **Weekly intermittent fasting**, which means restricting your eating on two or three non-consecutive days a week. Generally, you'll restrict your calorie intake by 60% or more, or to 500-600 calories. Some people advocate alternate-day fasting, but this is somewhat more aggressive and can make it difficult to get a balanced and adequate diet.

I practice weekly fasting every Monday, restricting my calorie intake to 500-600 (weekly intermittent fasting) and then practice time-restricted eating every few weeks, where I will eat for eight hours and fast for 16 hours, five days a week. At first I struggled with the hunger I had first thing in the morning before eating. But I soon got used to it and I now enjoy the many benefits of fasting. My memory feels much sharper, I don't get brain fog as much as I used to, and I am much less likely to experience that 'after-lunch slump' or symptoms of IBS.

Some medical practitioners will say that if you are going to practice intermittent fasting, then it is better to always have breakfast and have your fasting period later on, due to the benefits of eating a good, healthy breakfast. These benefits include boosting energy and brain power, getting those nutrients and minerals in first thing, and a lower chance of being overweight.

This 'gut R&R' could deliver benefits such as improved diversity of the microbiome, better gut barrier function and a healthier immune system.

I said the jury is still out, but there has been a lot of scholarly work on fasting over the last decade. Intermittent fasting of mice led to an increase in the volume of gut mucus (which is a good thing), and also helped the goblet cells which produce the mucus to do their job; it also increased the length of the villi, the little 'fingers' that make up the gut wall and help to absorb nutrients.

In another study, mice were put on a number of different regimes, as regards the type of food, the amount of calories, and whether food was available all day, or only once a day. The result was unexpected. Calorie count and healthy or unhealthy food made no difference to mouse life expectancy. However, mice who ate only once a day lived 11% longer than those who could eat at any time. Mice who ate once a day *and* ate a third less lived 28% longer than those who could eat what they liked. They also stayed healthier for longer.

Those are mice. We are people. Signing up a bunch of people to volunteer for intermittent fasting could be difficult. However, medical researchers have found that observant Muslims make a good source of subjects, since during the holy month of Ramadan they fast during sunlight hours, eating only after sunset and just before sunrise.

The Ramadan fast appears to help some people's gut health markedly, improving the diversity of microbiota in their gut. However, for people who have inflammatory bowel disease, it can make things worse. There's another catch, too: after Ramadan, the gut microbiome soon returns to what it was before. Intermittent fasting needs to be a continuous practice to work effectively as a maintenance program for gut health. It's not the kind of thing you can just switch on and off.

Why does it affect the microbiome? Because your gut is empty for a while if you adopt intermittent fasting, this helps the *Lachnospiraceae* bacteria, which live most happily in an empty gut. When you fast, other bacteria can't compete with them, so they can reproduce fast. *Lachnospiraceae* just happen to be important bacteria for producing butyrate, a short-chain fatty acid which helps send anti-inflammatory signals to your immune system.

Another bacteria, *Akkermansia muciniphila*, also rapidly grows when your gut is empty, and is associated with a decrease in intestinal inflammation. Like the *Lachnospiraeae*, *Akkermansia* can help improve the gut's barrier function, too. Other beneficial bacteria which are helped when intermittent fasting reduces the competition from other microbiota are *Prevotellaceae* and *Bacteroidetes*; both of these can help prevent or reduce obesity. Think of your gut as being like the sea, with its own tides. The gut microbiome changes with the tide – just as when walking the seashore at high tide, you'll see different life forms on the beach than you would at low tide.

Intermittent fasting may also help your digestive system in another way. The 'migrating motor complex' is a scientific way of describing the way your GI tract puts in a big squeeze every ninety minutes or so, a wave of contractions which pushes the contents of the gut down into the colon, cleaning out the gut like the streetcleaners after a parade. The migrating motor complex turns off when you eat, so if you are always 'grazing,' you don't leave it enough time to work.

Your gut also likes regular rhythms; it works out its own circadian rhythm. So if you work changing shifts, and move your meals around a lot, be aware that your gut's circadian rhythms could be getting out of sync.

Eating late in the evening is also unhelpful. That's because your insulin response is lower in the evening, so your blood sugar will stay high for a longer time than it would if you ate earlier. High blood sugar can increase your risk of type 2 diabetes, cardiovascular disease, and even stroke, so it's worth avoiding.

If you decide to adopt intermittent fasting, remember to keep it intermittent. If you basically go on hunger strike, your body will soon enter starvation mode. That will actually decrease the diversity of bacteria in your gut, and it can also prevent you losing weight.

Keeping a food journal will help you map your symptoms. For instance, if you had acid reflux three times last week, you may be able to see what the three meals preceding those events had in common. Food journaling also helps you to build healthy habits, as it's easy to compare pages and see where you have begun to drift away from your ideal diet towards easy choices or fast food. As well as helping with gut health, food journaling can help you lose weight, or can get you in form for a marathon run. Just having to write it all down makes you more mindful of what you are eating, and will tend to stop you snacking distractedly.

I would love to recommend you an app here to make your life easier. Unfortunately, most food journaling apps are very oriented towards calorie counting, which is not really the best use of a food journal. In fact, focusing on calories can lead to self-blaming and aggravate any tendency toward eating disorders.

Foods that you should always avoid

Some foods really ought not to be a part of your diet at all. Highly processed foods, in particular, are not healthful. Research repeatedly shows links between highly processed foods and 'bad' gut bacteria, or less diverse gut microbiomes.

Highly processed foods such as ready meals and sauces run a confidence trick on your healthy eating habits. You may think you're eating a healthy vegetable meal, but it's quite likely stuffed full of added sugar, salt and fat, as well as chemicals such as emulsifiers, preservatives, and colorings. It's also likely to contain saturated fats, rather than healthier fats like olive oil, groundnut oil, sesame oil, or sunflower oil (and palm oil, which is borderline, destroys rainforests and orangutan habitats – so if I see that on the label, the food doesn't go in my cart anyway).

Other highly processed foods that can be problematic include:

- Ham, salami, and other processed meats, which often contain high levels of salt as well as chemical additives.

- White bread, which is digested much faster than wholegrain bread, and so makes your blood sugar levels spike.

- Most snacks, as well as many breakfast cereals.

Highly processed foods are often made from ingredients that have already been highly processed themselves, such as whey, isolated proteins, corn syrups, and so on. But as well as including ingredients you don't want, they often miss out components that your digestion needs, such as fiber, protein, and healthy fats.

While most people know that processed foods contain too much salt and sugar, and not enough fiber, till recently there wasn't much research on what these foods do to your gut microbiome. But recent research shows they have a negative impact on the microorganisms in your GI tract. That's probably because a diet that's full of high-fat and high-sugar foods helps toxic bacteria reproduce faster.

On average, we eat half our daily calories in the form of highly processed foods. The higher the percentage of highly processed foods you eat, the more chances that you will become overweight or obese, or develop Type 2 diabetes. Highly processed foods have also been linked with increased cancer risks.

Refined carbs such as white rice, sugar and bread are often 'empty' calories, which include very few nutrients, with little fiber, vitamins or minerals left in them. They don't leave you feeling full for long; your blood sugar levels will suddenly drop after just an hour, whereas non-refined food would keep your blood sugar level for two or three hours. That means you'll want a snack sometime soon. If you keep cookies or potato chips in the house, you are just adding to the problem! That's why eating highly processed food can so quickly lead to putting on weight.

The most common highly processed foods to avoid are:

- Bacon, sausages, ham, paté, burgers.
- Baked beans, tinned spaghetti or ravioli.
- Ready-made sauces.
- Sodas, 'juice-based drinks.'
- Candies.
- Bakery products – cakes, muffins, white bread, cookies.
- Fast foods.
- Jams, sandwich spreads.
- Potato chips, pretzels, Pringles.
- Frozen meals, particularly pizza or pasta based.

You don't have to avoid them completely. A really nice piece of ham or salami every so often is fine. When I do buy paté, I get it from a butcher who makes it on the premises, from traceable, local meat – and as well as being healthier than supermarket products, it tastes a whole lot better too. Maybe have a burger when you go watch a football game with your friends. If you're out with the girls, fine, dip into the pretzels – but don't buy a packet to take home.

Sometimes it's best to find an alternative. Instead of using ready-sweetened oats for breakfast, use steel-cut oats and chop up a banana to go with them. Make your own flapjacks or traybakes instead of eating store-bought cookies, if you have time. Buy dried fruit without added sugar, or nuts and seeds, or just chop up a carrot, instead of snacking on potato chips.

Make your own salad dressing with a little olive oil and balsamic vinegar. I shake my own up in a small bottle, which really doesn't take much more time and is so much healthier than using salad cream or store-bought vinaigrette.

If you have more time, you might get interested in canning your own fruit and veg or drying your own fruit. I invested in a small fruit dryer, which uses only as much electricity as a light bulb and means I can make my own sweetener-free dried apple, tomato and so on.

AGEs

Advanced glycation end products (AGEs) are harmful compounds which can form in foods that have been exposed to very high temperatures, for instance by frying, grilling, or barbecuing. Fatty meat is particularly noted for producing AGEs, but cheese, butter, and oils can also do so. That means you might be eating healthy ingredients, but because you're cooking them at high temperatures, you're eating a lot of AGEs.

Your body can tolerate a certain amount of AGEs, because your digestive enzymes will cope. However, beyond that level, AGEs can become a problem. They can cause inflammation, and high levels of AGEs are linked to diseases such as diabetes and Alzheimer's, as well as heart disease. You're at particular risk if you also have high blood sugar levels.

Reducing AGEs is easy to do. Fry and grill less, for instance. If you scramble your eggs rather than frying them, you'll end up with sixteen times fewer AGEs; if you poach your chicken instead of frying it, you'll get 1,000 kilounits of AGEs per liter, against 5,200 if you grill the chicken. Try to find more recipes that involve slow cooking, such as stews, soups, and slow roasts; these produce fewer AGEs. One baked potato has a tenth the AGEs of the same amount of french fries.

You can also reduce AGEs by using the right ingredients. Cooking meat with acidic ingredients such as vinegar, lemon juice, or tomatoes can cut AGE production by half. Adding turmeric to meat can also help inhibit AGE production.

Cut down on red meat, which is a culprit both for AGEs and for inflammation, even if it's not highly processed. It also gives you too much omega-6 in relation to omega-3. Ideally, you'd want a two-to-one ratio. But a typical American diet delivers ten times more omega-6 than omega-3, and that's way out of whack. Concentrate on quality rather than quantity: one really good, lean steak once or twice a week rather than sausages or burgers every night. You'll get a lot of pleasure out of eating it, and you'll be healthier too.

Eating more fruit and vegetables and more wholegrains will help cut your AGEs and also keep you feeling full for longer.

Let's just talk a bit about the omegas, because although they are a relatively minor subject, they do have an impact. Omega-3 fatty acids help your GI tract stay healthy; in fact, they're essential for your body generally – and most Americans don't get enough of them. They are polyunsaturated fats and are anti-inflammatory, and you find them in three main food types:

1. Nuts and seeds; walnuts, flaxseeds, chia seeds have the highest omega-3 content, though other seeds like sunflower seed or pumpkin seed will also help. These are rich in alpha-linolenic acids (ALAs).

2. Seed oils including flaxseed oil, canola oil, perilla, walnut oil, and soy, all of which produce ALAs.

3. Oily fish – salmon, sardines, mackerel, tuna, and shellfish, trout, oysters, herring, and clams, which produce eicosapentoenoic acids (EPAs) and docosahexaenoic acids (DHAs).

Fish oils include EPA and DHA omega-3 fatty acids, which will do you good, but in fact, it's the ALAs you need most of, so adding nuts and seeds and their oils to your diet will help you the most.

Omega-3 does all kinds of good things, like reducing 'bad' cholesterol, feeding your brain, improving the health of your bones, hair and skin, and also plays a big role in gut health. It can help to decrease inflammation and increase the diversity of bacteria in your gut.

The good news? You only need to eat two portions of fatty fish every week to hit overall omega-3 targets, or you could take cod liver oil if you like. Adding anchovies to your diet can deliver a punch; try anchovy-stuffed olives, anchovy on top of your pizza, or chopped anchovies added to salad dressings to give a salty, fishy flavor.

You could use walnut oil in your salad dressings, or nibble walnuts as a snack; or you could add chia and flax seeds to your salad dressings and to breakfast muesli or porridge. Other oils also contain omega-3 fatty acids, but they add a lot of less-beneficial omega-6, which is why sunflower, corn, peanut and sesame oils are not as beneficial as walnut oil.

The problem of fats

It's quite common to see warnings telling people not to eat 'fatty' food. But actually, it's the *kind* of fat you are eating that will really affect your health.

There are three kinds of fats:

1.   Saturated fats.
2.   Unsaturated fats.
3.   Trans fats (technically, trans fatty acids).

Saturated fats, like milk, butter, and cheese, can raise 'bad' cholesterol. Meat, particularly fatty meat, contains saturated fat. Most vegetable foods don't, but coconut and palm oil are the exceptions.

Big sources of saturated fat in the average diet include pizzas, cheese, milk, butter, yogurts and other dairy-based desserts, meat products such as hamburgers, sausages, and bacon, cookies, and fast food.

Cutting back on saturated fats can be good for you, but only if you replace them with unsaturated fats. If you replace them with refined carbohydrates, that won't help.

Unsaturated fats are 'good' fats, which can help reduce your blood cholesterol levels; they are anti-inflammatory and can even help stabilize your heart rhythms. Unsaturated fats are found in olive oil and other plant oils (peanut, canola, sunflower, corn, soybean, flaxseed), in seeds (pumpkin, sesame, flax), and in nuts, as well as in fish and avocadoes and olives.

The worst kind of fats are the trans fats. These can be found naturally in small quantities, in beef and dairy fat, but mostly they come from the industrial creation of vegetable oils through hydrogenation. This process involves heating the oils up in the presence of hydrogen gas and a catalyst. It helps convert the fat into a solid, like margarine, allows the oil to be reheated numerous times, and stops it becoming rancid.

Fast food restaurants love trans fats for frying, while a lot of processed snack foods are fried with trans fats or include large amounts of trans fats in the ingredients. When you see a food label that includes the words 'hydrogenated vegetable oil,' that's the trans fat content.

Trans fats don't just add 'bad' cholesterol, as saturated fats do. They also reduce 'good' cholesterol (HDL), an unhealthy double whammy. So it's worth always *checking* that your oil or shortening doesn't contain hydrogenated oils.

Foods that cause bloating

Almost a third of people experience a feeling of bloatedness from time to time, some of them quite often. There are a number of foods that cause bloating, so it is well worth cutting them out of your diet to see if that helps.

Beans are a particularly bad food for flatulence and bloating. They do have lots of fiber and vitamins, which is good. But they can really make your life uncomfortable because they belong to the FODMAPs group. Soak your beans or eat beansprouts instead of beans, and they're a bit easier for your system to handle.

Lentils, again, are basically a really healthy food containing plenty of fiber, protein, and carbs; but you guessed it, they also belong to the FODMAPs group. As with beans, if you sprout or soak lentils well before you cook, it can lower the bloat factor.

Green vegetables are good for you, but again, there are some which can give you gas or bloating: broccoli, cabbage, and Brussels sprouts. Replace those with spinach, cucumbers, lettuce, and zucchini and see if it does you good.

Onions contain fructans and could bloat you or give you gas. Jain people don't eat onions or garlic (or other root vegetables), yet Jain cooking is very tasty thanks to the subtle use of herbs and spices. So if you want to give up onions, take a tip from them and use herbs and spices to replace the flavor, or other tasty additions such as the green part of scallions.

Wheat and rye can be replaced with alternatives like quinoa, oats, buckwheat, sorghum flour, rice flour, or brown rice. If you can't find these things in the supermarket, try a health food shop, which will often have a good variety of gluten-free and other unusual foods.

Believe it or not, if you have IBS, an apple a day might not keep the doctor away, due to the high amount of fructose, which is a FODMAP. You could eat your apples cooked rather than raw, which can help, or try eating bananas, berries, or citrus fruits instead.

Beer can be a bloat-inducer too, as it contains gluten, is often carbonated, and contains fermentable carbs. You could drink wine or spirits instead. If you're a craft beer fan, of course, this may not be good news. However, many breweries are now making exceptionally good gluten-free beers, which might be worth trying to see if they help with the problem.

SWEETENERS

Artificial sweeteners sounded like a fantastic idea. You could replace all that 'bad,' calorie-rich sugar with 'good,' calorie-free sweeteners. Well, things haven't quite turned out that way. Sweeteners are really not good for you at all.

An Israeli study showed that just two weeks of using artificial sweetener changed the gut flora of mice – and that made them obese. This was then followed up by a trial in humans which showed similar results. Out of the various sweeteners available, sucralose, aspartame and saccharin are particularly bad, and can even lead eventually to glucose intolerance. Another study showed that the use of sweeteners could increase the ability of *E.coli* and *E.faecalis* to attack the intestinal lining. In other words, if you put sweetener in your coffee, you're increasing the likelihood of serious digestive trouble.

You may think you don't take sweeteners, but again, a spot of label-checking might show you that you ingest more than you think. They're in your toothpaste! And lipstick! And even in vitamin capsules! So be sure to read the small print.

Natural sweeteners that are okay include xylitol, a sugar alcohol, which actually supports a good microbiome in your gut. Yacon syrup, from a South American plant, is also beneficial, with plenty of soluble fiber to feed beneficial bacteria in your digestive tract. But go gently – both these sweeteners can cause bloating and gas if you take too much. Some people suggest licorice root as another natural sweetener that can help, but the jury's out on that one.

If you use canned fruit in cooking, choose fruit that's packed in juice, not syrup. Add fresh fruit or dried fruit (sultanas, dried cranberries or apricot) to recipes to replace sugars, and use more almond or vanilla essence in recipes to add taste without adding sugar.

Fiber

Fiber is 'roughage' which doesn't get broken down in your small intestine. It passes through your large intestine pretty much intact, and bulks out your stool, preventing constipation. Insoluble fiber such as whole-wheat flour, wheat bran, nuts, beans, potatoes and cauliflower promotes movement of material through your GI tract, keeping you 'regular.'

Soluble fiber, on the other hand, dissolves in water to form a gel. This can help to lower your cholesterol and glucose levels. Soluble fiber is found in oats, peas, beans, apples, citrus, carrots, and barley.

For best results, you want a mix of fibers, and it's also best if that fiber is contained in real food, rather than fiber supplements. So, for instance, you could start eating a high-fiber breakfast cereal, like bran, or have wholegrain instead of white toast. Remember, the more refined a food is, the less fiber it contains; brown rice has much more fiber than white rice. For main meals, you could use brown rice or bulgur wheat, and add pulses such as lentils, peas, kidney beans or black beans to your meal. You could also add oatmeal to cake and cookie recipes, and snack on fresh or dried fruit.

High fiber can normalize your bowel movements, but fiber-rich food is also very filling, so that can help you reduce weight by keeping you from feeling peckish. Don't forget to drink plenty of water so the fiber is well hydrated.

It's best to introduce more fiber into your diet gradually, rather than try to make an instant change. You might also want to introduce one high-fiber food at a time, as some foods with plenty of fiber may not work well for you personally. For instance, chickpeas and cereals tend to trigger my IBS, so I avoid them. I make up my fiber elsewhere.

Generally, if you have IBS, you'll benefit from tailoring your diet to include more *soluble* fiber. Psyllium supplements can be useful, as it doesn't get broken down by your digestive system too fast, and so doesn't create a lot of gas. Linseed and flaxseed are also good sources of fiber for IBS sufferers, ground or whole; make sure you take them with a good glassful of water.

You may also need to allow for a short period of disturbance, because you're changing your habits, before the fiber starts to help you.

Foods that give you plenty of soluble fiber include avocados, apples, pears, strawberries, blueberries, sweet potatoes, carrots, turnips, peas, oats, beans, bran and barley.

Reading the small print

If you see something on a label you don't recognize, it probably isn't great for your health. In fact, generally, the fewer ingredients on a label, the better. If I buy a chicken salad and the label says 'lettuce, tomatoes, chicken, vinegar, olive oil, arugula,' I'm happy. But imagine you buy a chicken salad and the ingredients list looks like this:

- Chicken, water, manioc starch, salt, modified vinegar, sugars (cultured dextrose, corn syrup solids), sodium phosphate, carrageen (maltodextrin, potassium chloride), yeast extract, lemon juice powder, sunflower oil, calcium silicate, xanthan gum.

- Mayonnaise – canola oil, liquid whole egg and liquid yolk, water, vinegar, salt, sugar, spices, concentrated lemon juice, calcium disodium edta, citric acid.

- Celery, sour cream (modified milk ingredients, cornstarch, bacterial culture, carob bean gum, sodium citrate, onion, spices).

That's from the label on a Costco chicken salad. I spot a few words there I don't like. 'Cultured' and 'modified' for instance. There are lots of processed ingredients: the lemon juice is concentrated or comes as a powder; it didn't come straight from pressing a lemon. And there's sugar in the mayonnaise. When I make chicken salad at home, this is what goes in it: chicken, mayonnaise (egg, olive oil, white wine vinegar, Dijon mustard), celery, lettuce. Seven ingredients, tops.

Watch out for natural sugars. White sugar is sucrose, a nutrient-free processed food with a lot of calories. But you'll also find:

- Fructose, in fruits, carrots, and honey.

- Glucose, in carbohydrates.

- Galactose, in dairy and avocados.

- Lactose, in milk (glucose + galactose = lactose).

- Maltose, produced out of the starch in barley, wheat and corn, and also found in peaches and pears.

If you eat too much sugar, the small intestine can't process it all. If it reaches the large intestine, pathogenic bacteria will use it. Most of us in developed western countries eat four to five times more sugar than we ought to – one can of Coke has more sugar than the recommended daily intake for an adult.

In fact, you're probably not going to eat too much sugar if you stick to fruits, avocados and grains. But watch out for it in processed foods; dextrose, dextrin, nectar, caramel, syrup, diastase, maltol, and mannose are all likely to mean added sugar.

Natural and organic

'Natural,' by the way, doesn't always mean better or healthier. For instance, although some herbs are fantastic remedies, not all are; echinacea doesn't seem to have any benefit against catching colds, for instance.

Some plants can be dangerous, like deadly nightshade (the name should give you a hint). Kava, a plant from Polynesia, is sometimes used as a supplement to treat anxiety, but it's also been linked to liver damage.

And often, 'natural' is used as a kind of whitewash, a piece of marketing jargon. Meat can be labeled 'natural' but still be pumped full of growth hormones. A dessert can be full of corn syrup but as long as it doesn't use any artificial sweeteners or colorings, it's 'natural.' A fruit or vegetable is 'natural' but could have been grown with lots of chemical fertilizers and pesticides, which may have left residue on the skin.

'Organic,' on the other hand, does give you some guarantees, and personally I far prefer to find organic food – it's better for the environment as well as for your gut. Specific certifications differ, and the label will show you the body which certifies the food, so you can look up exactly what it involves. Some governments have regulations in place to determine what is organic; in the US, farmers must use the USDA Organic label unless they sell less than $5,000 worth of organic product a year (that exemption means local gardeners or farmers with a limited production of veg and fruit can sell their organic veg without having to get certified).

For processed foods, the term 'organic' can only be used if all the ingredients, or at least 95% of them are organic. 'Made with organic' means that 70% or more of the ingredients are organic, e.g. 'made with organic oats,' and if this is the case, the ingredient list must show which ingredients are organic. Some voluntary labels may be even more strict.

Organic food can cost more; many organic producers are relatively small, so they don't get economies of scale, and production is often more labor-intensive.

If you can't afford organic, or don't have any local stores that offer organic produce, then try to buy the vegetables that are grown with the lowest amounts of pesticides. The table below shows which fruit and veg are usually grown without much pesticide, and those which are typically grown using high amounts of pesticide. You might choose to buy organic versions of the 'dirty dozen,' which will cut down your exposure dramatically, and buy regular produce from the low-pesticide group. Also try to buy organic if you're eating the skin, for instance apples and grapes, or for leaf vegetables like spinach and kale.

A really good way to get organic food is to grow your own, if you have a balcony, a windowsill or a garden. It's time consuming, but really worthwhile.

For meat, buying organic means the animals have had access to pasture, and the meat is hormone free, which will give you higher levels of omega-3 fatty acids as well as improved taste.

Low pesticide use	High pesticide use – the 'dirty dozen'
Sweetcorn	Strawberries
Avocado	Apples
Pineapple	Nectarines
Cabbage	Peaches
Onion	Celery
Frozen peas	Grapes
Papaya	Cherries
Asparagus	Spinach
Mango	Tomatoes
Eggplant	Bell peppers
Melon	Cherry tomatoes
Kiwi fruit	Cucumbers
Cauliflower	
Grapefruit	

Pesticides are widely used in non-organic agriculture to destroy bugs, weeds, rats, fungi, mildew and moulds. Synthetic pesticides are created in labs; several types have now been banned, such as many organophosphates (targeting the nervous system of insects) and some neocotinoids (insecticide that can kill whole colonies of bees).

Organic pesticides are made from plants, but they are not always trouble-free. For instance, rotenone is produced by a number of tropical plants as a beetle deterrent. You might think that would be safe to use, but if it gets into watercourses, it's toxic to fish.

You're protected by legal limits on the amount of pesticide that can be used; however, the European Union says nearly 3% of food samples contained pesticide levels above the legally permitted amounts, and a Canadian report found over 1%. There is still, then, a small risk.

To get rid of pesticides:

- Wash fruit and veg with water, which should get rid of 60-70% of residues.

- Peel potatoes, carrots, etc. (though this destroys a lot of the extra nutrients that are found in the skin).

- Shop at farmers' markets where you know the food meets organic standards!

Get in tune with your body

One big benefit of keeping a 'food and mood' diary is that as you get used to writing about how you feel, and how your digestion feels, you'll get more in tune with your body.

You'll get to have a feel for the kind of foods that affect your system. It may be only one or two foods, or it may be a whole group of foods such as dairy or gluten.

Intolerance	Allergy
Affects your digestion	Affects your immune system
Causes digestive problems	Can cause major allergic reactions – shortness of breath, rashes, swelling
Symptoms occur a few hours after eating	Symptoms occur at once
You're probably okay to eat a little bit of a food to which you're intolerant	Even the smallest quantity can cause a life-threatening reaction

If you find you're intolerant to particular foods, you may need to change your diet – not just to cut them out, but to find another source of the nutrients they deliver. If you can't eat gluten, your fiber intake will go down, so you'll need to replace it with food from other food groups.

You'll also find out how much food is right for you. A lot of us regularly overeat. Fill up on lean proteins and non-starchy veg and fruit first, and you may not even have an appetite for high-carb/high-fat foods after that. Keeping a food diary will show how much you *really* eat, not how much you think you're eating.

Watch out for dopamine effects. High fat, salt or sugar content can activate pleasure centers in your brain which can override your feelings of satiety, so you eat too much, even though you're full. Dole out smaller portions to stop getting a sugar high; if you feel dozy after eating, you probably had too much. Paying more attention to how you feel while you're eating and after you've eaten will really help you work out what to eat, and how much of it.

You may want to change some of your habits. We all get into habits, and when they're really ingrained, we sometimes fail to even realize they're there. Your food diary will show you exactly what habits you have, as you reflect on your eating over the week. Do you always need a sugary snack mid-afternoon? Do you always feel sleepy after lunch? Do you skip meals?

Your food diary can also help you work out why you have these bad habits. Is it stress or boredom that made you eat that chocolate? Or you may be a victim of circumstances. Hotel buffet breakfasts can be a terrible thing, as you keep going back for more. Or a plate full of donuts at a team meeting might be irresistible (hint: you can move the donut plate up the table, away from you!).

Once you've taken a look at your food diary, you can then choose what things you want to fix first. Can you avoid the cues and the triggers for some of your bad habits? I still have hotel buffet breakfasts, but now I start off loading up with oats and nuts. Then if I *still* feel a bit hungry, I might have something else.

Find some new good habits. One of my friends downloaded a Hare Krishna cookbook and made every dish in it over a couple of months. She now has loads of healthy, tasty, vegetarian dishes that she knows how to make. The challenge of cooking these dishes, she says, also took her mind off the craving for chocolate. I know several people who have taken up meal prepping so they always have a healthy meal ready ahead of time, and all they need to do is heat it up. Other good habits are:

GOOD HABITS

- Pay attention to your food. Don't watch TV while you're eating.
- Don't eat when you're not really hungry. Don't eat more when you feel full.
- If you eat too fast, then put your fork down between mouthfuls (this is sneaky, and it works).
- Don't go to the store hungry!

Eat mindfully

Some families still say a prayer before meals (though one French friend told me, "I know why the English say prayers before meals. It's because they're eating English food!"). It's a good idea, whether you believe in a deity or not, to have a moment of stillness and calm before you start eating. Take a few deep breaths, let your body relax, and breathe out all the stress and tension of the day.

Experience your different hungers. There's desperate growly hunger when you get home late and have had nothing since an inadequate lunch. There's "I think I ought to be eating because it's lunchtime" hunger. There's emotional hunger, when you feel sad or stressed and want to eat. There are cravings. And then you might feel hungry because you just smelt a whiff of stew heating up, or you heard a barbecue sizzling.

Sometimes, what you experience as 'hunger' is actually thirst. Try drinking half a glass of water. Do you still feel as hungry as you did?

Emotional hunger might really be asking you to slow down or de-stress, rather than eat. Go for a walk outside and see if that fits the bill.

Pay attention to the food with all your senses – how it looks, the texture of the food, how it smells and tastes, even the sound – does it crunch when you bite it, or sizzle on the plate? You may even find emotions and memories come back when you're eating, particularly if you're eating a dish you were fond of as a child.

Chew your food. Don't just swallow it; chew it a good few times and savor it.

Cut out addictive foods while you're trying to change your habits. A little voice screaming "chocolate!" is difficult to ignore. But if you cut chocolate out for a couple of weeks, you can pay more attention to what you're actually eating. You may find that your body is saying, "Hey, I really love melon" or "It's avocado time!" Finding new foods that you love, and that are good for you, is a fantastic result.

Spend a few moments after you've eaten reflecting on the meal. Was it nourishing? Too little? Too much? Was it tasty? Maybe too tasty? Or not enough? Does it leave you feeling good?

Don't beat yourself up. Habits take a while to develop or change. Don't think "I just blew the whole diet" if you succumbed to one small craving; that's perfectly normal, early on. Give yourself a little love; think again about why you're changing that habit. Don't be the bad schoolteacher who kept telling you that you'd never amount to anything, that you'd never pass your exams or get a decent job. Be the nice schoolteacher who gave you seven out of ten and then said "but I know you can do better next time."

Try to become more mindful of how your body feels generally, and not just around food. For instance, in the morning, wake up by gently asking each part of your body how it feels. Then stretch, and relax, and see how you're feeling. *Now* you're ready to get up.

If you always feel your shoulders ache, you've got tension there that you need to let go of. If you feel tight, then loosen your body by gently shaking or wiggling your arms and legs, maybe flopping over a couple of times as if you're touching your toes (don't force it, just let yourself flop), and very gently rotating your head to relax your neck. Try to ensure you don't start eating when you're feeling tense, even if it means waiting another couple of minutes.

Here's one thing I'll add from my own experience: if you're trying to change your diet, don't try to 'fake' what you ate before. I find most gluten-free bread is just horrible. So I prefer to have a quinoa salad with my lunch, rather than gluten-free bread, and if I feel hungry, I'll have a handful of sunflower seeds and pumpkin seeds, not a cookie. Also, if you try something different, you're going to think, "Wow, I'm trying all this new stuff! Some of it is really tasty!" rather than "I'm not allowed to eat all these things that I used to." It's a much more positive approach.

Hopefully while reading this chapter you've realized that adjusting your diet isn't quite as simple as it sounds. You need to find the right foods for your gut, but at the same time give the rest of your body the nutrients that it needs, so there will inevitably be some give and take involved. Fortunately, for most of us it's a trade-off between which foods irritate our GI tract a bit and which foods we really need or aren't prepared to do without (I suspect for many of us, chocolate is on the 'can't do without' list).

Keeping a food diary will really help you find out which foods have the worst effect on your gut, and which foods are tolerable.

The action steps for this chapter are really just carrying out what we've been talking about.

ACTION STEPS

1. Decide on the scope of your elimination diet: whether you want to eliminate a particular group, or all the potentially troublesome foods.

2. Plan a month when you don't have too much travel or stress involved, and can carry out the elimination diet without too many other factors getting in the way.

3. Start your food diary in advance of the diet, for best results. This gives you a 'control' that you can look back to and see whether the elimination diet is making a difference.

4. Eliminate!

5. Start adding the foods back and noting the ones that lead to flare-ups or cause you to feel depressed or lethargic. Let your diet settle down, continue with the diary, and check that you're still getting a good, balanced diet. Life is better, I hope!

Nourish Your Gut, Share the Glow

Embrace the Gift of Wellness

"True wealth is health—share it generously" - Hippocrates

People who share wellness without expecting anything in return live longer, happier lives. So let's spread the glow together.

I've got a question for you, a chance to be a guiding light for someone who needs it most. Imagine a person like you, or maybe the version of you before the transformation. Eager to make a difference but uncertain where to look for gut health wisdom.

Our mission is to make gut health accessible to everyone. Every word in Gut Health Secrets for Women stems from that mission. And to make it happen, I need to reach... well... everyone.

This is where your generosity can shine. Most folks do judge a book by its cover and reviews. So here's my ask on behalf of a searching soul in the realm of gut health:

Could you take a moment to leave a review for Gut Health Secrets for Women?

How You Can Help:

1. Scan the QR code below to leave your review on Amazon.
2. Share your thoughts and let others know how this book can guide them to enhance their gut health.

Your gift costs nothing but a minute of your time, yet it could alter a fellow wellness seeker's life. Your review might...

- Help someone retore their gut health.
- Help someone learn good diet habits for a healthy gut.
- Empower someone to transform their life.

- Bring one more dream to life.

To experience that heart-warming feeling and genuinely make a difference, all you have to do is... in less than 60 seconds... leave a review.

Scan the QR code below to leave your review (just so you know, this takes you to the review page of Amazon US, if you live in a different country, simply change the .com to the relevant country domain suffix. Or you can go to your order page to leave a review there):

If the idea of helping an anonymous wellness seeker resonates with you, welcome to the club. You're one of us.

I'm thrilled to support you in achieving your wellness goals faster, easier, and more joyfully than you can imagine. The upcoming chapters are filled with tactics, lessons, and strategies that you'll love.

Thank you from the depths of my heart.

Your biggest supporter, Naomi

PS - Did you know? Providing value to others makes you more valuable to them. If you think this book can help another wellness seeker, share the glow and send it their way.

Chapter 6
DETOX AND RESET

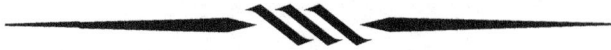

H ave you ever wished you could reboot your body as easily as you can reboot a computer? Well, that's what a detox is – a body reboot.

There are plenty of good reasons to detox:

- You can increase your energy levels with the right mix of foods.

- You can get rid of inflammation by eliminating pro-inflammatory food groups like gluten, dairy and sugar.

- You're supporting your digestive system with light foods and high fiber.

- A detox can boost your immune system.

- A detox can clear up your skin.

- You can lose weight and speed up your metabolism.

- You can improve your sleep.

- You can reset your tastebuds!

- You can reset your emotions!

But let me add a warning. Many popular detox diets are just fads. You need to be careful to check out a detox program and ensure you're not missing out on good nutrition, or a detox could make things worse rather than better.

Colon cleansing is one of those fads. There's only one time you really need colonic irrigation, and that's if you're having a colonoscopy tomorrow. Basically, it's like an enema, only more thorough. It's based on the idea that toxins and waste build up in your colon, and you need to clean it out.

There's only one problem: there is no scientific evidence at all for this. In fact, natural bacteria in your colon detoxify food waste as part of your digestive system, while mucous membranes in the colon stop toxins entering your bloodstream; and most calories and nutrients are absorbed by the GI tract before they hit the large intestine. Plus there's the 'big wave' of migrating motor complex to clear things out periodically. So if your digestive system is working properly, your colon is already clean.

Colonic irrigation brings a number of risks with it: dehydration, cramps, nausea, bacterial imbalance or infection, and depletion of your natural gut bacteria. Coffee enemas are a particularly bad idea; it's a waste of good coffee, but more seriously, coffee enemas can lead to a severe allergic reaction. And your digestive system is delicate – do you really want to go sticking things up there?

The risk of side effects increases if you have hemorrhoids, Crohn's disease, or ulcerative colitis.

A better way to flush the system is to take plenty of fiber. It's like getting lots of little scouring pads to tumble down your large intestine, cleaning it as they go, and you'll just be helping your natural gut microbiome do its job, rather than interfering with it.

Superfoods

Superfoods can provide you with a natural detox. For instance, spirulina is 65% protein, contains all the nine essential amino acids, as well as B and E vitamins, zinc, manganese, selenium, copper and iron. It's a good protein source if you are vegan or vegetarian, and it's rich in iron, which is good news if you have ever suffered from anemia. It also contains phycocyanin, which helps new blood cells to grow, and chlorophyll, which is similar to hemoglobin and is a good blood purifier.

Spirulina can help decrease your blood pressure, as it helps increase the production of nitric oxide, which dilates and relaxes the blood vessels. It's a good source of calcium too, so if you're on a non-dairy diet, can help replace the lost calcium from milk products. It's high in antioxidants, which help protect from toxins such as cancers, and it can even help eliminate heavy metals and arsenic from the system.

What's the downside of spirulina? It tastes absolutely vile. My advice: take the tablets, not the powder.

Other superfoods include spinach, blueberries, kale, arugula (rocket), and broccoli. They're full of antioxidants, vitamins A, C, and E, and they are great for your skin and hair.

In fact, just about any green veg is good for you. Have a green vegetable detox by just making sure you have a big portion of green veg once a day, whatever it is. Find greens you love; for me, that's kale, Chinese leaf, arugula and spinach, and pak choi if I can get it. Arugula is particularly great because you can use it as a topping for any dish, add it to salad, or even make pesto with it, and the peppery taste will spice up the blandest meal.

Cabbage and kale are very good for you. I don't personally rate the 'cabbage soup diet,' as it excludes too many foods, and it's also boring; but eating plenty of cabbage is a good idea. Kimchi and sauerkraut are great foods, as they add the probiotic strength of fermented foods to the goodness of cabbage. These vegetables have anti-inflammatory properties; they also contain glutathione, which promotes liver function, and sulforaphane, which protects from cancer and toxins.

Asparagus is a natural diuretic. Rather than boiling it, roast it in the oven drizzled with a little olive oil, to keep all the flavor in. Asparagus also provides the antioxidant glutathione, along with fiber, iron, and vitamins

A, C, E, and K.

HERE ARE SOME GREAT GREEN SUPERFOODS TO TRY:

- Basil, which you can use as a dressing or in salad, to make pesto, or as an infusion. Basil reduces water retention.
- Broccoli maintains your blood sugar level, is an antioxidant, and fights infection; steamed, boiled, or roasted, but leave it just a bit crunchy to get the best out of it.
- Lemongrass can be used in tea, or in Asian cooking.
- Mint is great added to tea or to drinking water, and in salads, and goes well with feta cheese and courgettes.
- Cilantro deals with mercury in the body, and is said to prevent urinary tract infections. It's great used as a topping or in a salsa.
- Beet greens are used in southern Italian cooking as a regular green vegetable, for instance in pasta sauce.
- Beetroot can be eaten raw, juiced, boiled, in salad or in soup. It's a super detox choice, as it lowers bad cholesterol and purifies the blood and liver.
- Wheatgrass is good for you, and provides 70% of its weight in chlorophyll; just add a little to smoothies. You don't need a whole lot.
- Bok choy/pak choy is one of my favorite vegetables, and is great in a stir fry, or braised. If you like your greens crunchy, pak choy stems are fantastic.
- Watercress, mustard greens and chicory are also really flavorsome additions to your green veg lineup.

Be careful not to eat too much spinach, swiss chard and beet greens, as they have high amounts of oxalic acid, which can deplete the calcium in your bones. Eating them twice a week is probably enough, or just scatter a few leaves in your salads. If you cook them with cream, butter, seeds, nuts, or coconut oil, that can help to counterbalance the oxalic acid.

Don't overboil your green veg. Blanching (cooking very quickly in already boiling water, and then rinsing in ice cold water straight away to preserve the green color), steaming, stir-frying or roasting are better than boiling for keeping all the vitamins as well as all the flavor.

If you are bored with salads, by the way, just jazz up the dressings. For instance, you could mix tahini and miso with lemon juice and a little warm water, or blitz a couple of fresh strawberries into your vinaigrette. Fruit-flavored balsamic vinegars can also be a great store-cupboard purchase, as they bring a zing to your salad.

ANTIOXIDANTS

Free radicals are highly unstable molecules which are formed when you digest or exercise, and can also be acquired from cigarette smoke or polluted air. They can trigger cell damage and may be at the root of many cancers. Antioxidants attach the free radicals together, making them stable and harmless – a bit like a big glob of putty that dust and dirt will stick to.

The science is unclear on the exact mechanisms at work. Antioxidant *supplements* apparently don't decrease the likelihood of developing various diseases, with one exception: a combination of antioxidants do lower the risk of developing age-related macular degeneration (AMD), a disease that can lead to blindness in later life. There are various large studies on this: in-depth information can be found at https://www.nccih. nih.gov/health/antioxidants-in-depth. But antioxidant-rich vegetables *do* appear to maintain health, through decreasing oxidative stress that can contribute to chronic diseases such as Alzheimer's and various cancers. This may be because they include a much higher diversity of components – for instance, eight forms of vitamin E instead of typically just one in supplements.

Green tea is not actually a green vegetable, but it's still good for your detox, particularly if you use it to replace black tea or coffee. It contains lots of antioxidants, and helps hydration. Increasing your fluid intake can help weight loss, and green tea can help burn fat faster. Incorporate it as part of your general diet. If, like me, you actually like the taste, so much the better! The downside is that it contains caffeine, though not so much as black tea. Green tea infusions with lemon, strawberry, ginger, vanilla, or mint, can be really refreshing.

You might also make dandelion tea. Dandelion leaves are packed with vitamins A, B, C, and E, zinc, calcium, magnesium, potassium, and manganese iron. Boil them for five minutes to make a diuretic tea which will help to flush out your system (make sure you're drinking enough water to replace the lost liquid). Or you could mix a few leaves into a salad – they are slightly bitter, so don't use too many.

Lemon is a rich source of vitamin C, provides antioxidants, and is good for your skin. During detox, take warm water with lemon juice as a morning drink, and add just a dash of lemon juice to the water you drink with a meal, hot or cold. Add a little ginger if you like.

Another citrus superfood is grapefruit. It contains tons of nutrients: vitamins A, B1, and C, fiber, potassium, biotin, and enzymes that can help break down food. If you want to lose weight, grapefruit is a good friend.

Ginger is a superfood, and recognized as such in Ayurvedic medicine. An infusion of root ginger ('ginger tea') is a great tonic and can help reduce flatulence and bloating. If you cook Asian-influenced recipes, they will usually include plenty of root ginger. By the way, many sailors swear by ginger (often in the form of 'ginger nut' biscuits) as a way to counteract seasickness, so if you feel nauseous, ginger can help.

Brown rice is the fiber of choice for detox. It will give you vitamin B, manganese, phosphorus, and high levels of fiber, which will help keep your colon clean with no recourse to artificial methods.

DETOX SMOOTHIE

You don't need to pay for supplements, protein powders, or energy drinks if you want to undergo a thorough detox. This smoothie provides a 100% fruit and veg reboot for your system.

Ingredients:

- Half a cup of orange juice.
- A green apple.
- Half a cup pineapple.
- Half a banana.
- Half an inch of root ginger.
- A cup of fresh spinach.
- A handful of cilantro (coriander leaf).
- A tablespoon of lime juice.

Mince the ginger, core the apple, and blitz the spinach, cilantro and ginger; then add the fruit and blitz it coarsely, and your smoothie is ready.

Why these ingredients? Green apple has a lower sugar content than riper apples, but has just as much pectin, which is a prebiotic. Pineapple is rich in antioxidants, and contains a protein-digesting enzyme that can help your digestion (that's why some marinades for meat contain pineapple juice). Banana gives you potassium, which lowers blood pressure and can help with muscle cramps, while ginger is anti-inflammatory. Spinach is full of antioxidants, while cilantro is thought to combat heavy metal toxicity, but more importantly, tastes good; and finally, the lime gives you another jolt of vitamin C.

Take this first thing and you may well find you'll feel full for longer, and eat better for the rest of the day, too.

Something that's become pretty modish recently is the apple cider vinegar detox. That involves drinking a mix of two tablespoons of unfiltered apple cider vinegar, eight ounces of water, and a drop of honey or stevia, with lemon juice, or chili, or cayenne pepper. An actor friend uses it with plenty of chili, honey and lemon juice if she has a cold during a run of performances. It frees her throat and vocal cords up for a couple of hours so she can do her job.

It's a great idea. Apple cider vinegar is actually good for you. But will it detox your body?

It will give you a good dose of enzymes and can support your immune system and digestion. It can also add some good bacteria to your gut microbiome. There are a few results from small studies that show there may be benefits in terms of weight loss, lower cholesterol levels, and preventing atherosclerosis (the buildup of fats, cholesterol and other substances in and on the artery walls), but they're not conclusive. It may also reduce the rise in your blood sugar after a meal, and can promote the breakdown of fats, too, particularly 'bad' cholesterols. The main downside appears to be that it can make you feel slightly nauseous and cause indigestion in some people. Be careful not to drink it on a regular basis, as it can damage tooth enamel. If you're diabetic, discuss with your doctor if you want to start drinking it.

However, the detox is mixed with water. Do not, under any circumstances, drink apple cider vinegar undiluted!

Some doctors question whether detoxes are needed at all. The liver is meant to do that job for us – but of course, it relies on good gut health, as it's linked to your digestive system. The liver is your own natural detox system. Are there foods that are good for your liver? The answer is yes: all citrus fruits will help the liver produce the right enzymes, as will broccoli and cauliflower, which also contain sulfur compounds that keep your liver healthy.

Other good liver-aiding foods include:

- Garlic, which has selenium in it.

- Turmeric, which boosts bile production.
- Artichokes, which also help bile production and contain a wide variety of nutrients.
- Beets, which contain betaine (helps the liver get rid of toxins).
- Avocado, which is nutrient dense.
- Cabbage, which contains glutathione, an antioxidant that helps improve the liver's detoxifying functions.
- Green tea, which can protect against fatty liver disease.

Glutathione is a really powerful antioxidant, and one that the body makes itself (endogenously). It binds all the toxins it finds together, so that they can then be removed from the body, and it's detoxing you 24/7, all year round. So it's vital for liver health. Unfortunately, we make less and less of it as we grow older, and if you drink alcohol, your glutathione levels could fall.

What can help is eating foods – and maybe taking supplements – that can encourage your body to produce more glutathione. Grapefruit, apples, oranges, bananas, broccoli, peaches, melon, watercress, horseradish, turnips, cauliflower, Brussels sprouts, kale, peppers and squash will all increase the activity of the GST enzymes that help glutathione do its job.

A supplement that can help is NAC (N-acetyl-cysteine), which is a building block for glutathione; it's used in medical emergency detoxes for overdoses. To support this, you could also take folate and vitamins B6 and B12. Folate helps to ensure the cysteine prioritizes glutathione production rather than other processes; both B6 and B12 are necessary for the body to synthesize glutathione.

Staying hydrated

Staying hydrated is always important, but particularly when you're detoxing. The human body is nearly two-thirds water, and it evaporates all the time, through sweat, through vapor in our breath, and every time we use the bathroom. Our bodies work through fluids – digesting, absorbing, circulating. Water in your body, like a car radiator, keeps you from overheating. You need saliva to chew and swallow easily, and to make food more digestible when it reaches your stomach.

Water helps your kidneys do their job. The main toxin they remove is blood urea nitrogen; this is water-soluble, and the kidneys turn it to urine so that it can be expelled. If your urine is too dark in color, it means you're dehydrated. This put you at risk of getting kidney stones if you don't drink enough.

Water also helps your bowels stay regular. You're most likely to get constipated when you don't drink enough, and your body pulls water away from your digestive system.

So, drinking plenty of water is good for your digestion. But the 'eight glasses a day' guideline is something of a myth. That's the total liquid you need; it doesn't have to be water. If you eat a lot of water-containing foods like melon and cucumber, that will deliver liquid too. However, water is the easiest way to make sure you're staying properly hydrated.

A good guideline is to have a cool water bottle at hand and drink whenever you're thirsty. Make sure that you drink with every meal, too. When you have a break, choose a drink that you like, such as a herbal or fruit infusion, or green tea. In summer, make a cold tea in advance. I particularly like karkadeh, a hibiscus tea that's very popular in Egypt; you can get hibiscus tea at most good tea and coffee shops.

A bonus if you want to lose weight is that drinking water, and eating foods with a high water content, can make you feel full, so you'll probably eat less. Soups and stews can add extra water to your diet.

Alcoholic drinks don't count though. Alcohol can actually make you *lose* liquid from your body. And watch out for black tea, coffee and some herb infusions, which work as diuretics – again, you'll be losing more liquid than you take in.

Liquid intake needs to be coordinated with exercise, as muscles get fatigued when they don't have adequate fluids. Drink two hours before you exercise, and keep drinking while you exercise, particularly if it's hot.

What not to eat and drink during a detox

Alcohol is a big no when you're detoxing. So is caffeine, so that means no coffee and no black tea (green tea does contain caffeine, but in much lower amounts, and it offers certain health benefits, so that's fine as a part of your detox).

Excluding meat helps. You will detox best if you become vegetarian for the duration.

Processed and packaged foods ought to be left out. That includes frozen foods that have artificial ingredients added. Dairy, with the exception of kefir, is also a no-go area, and it can be a great idea to miss gluten out, particularly wheat.

Finally, cut out as much sugar as possible. Don't add sugar to your drinks or muesli, for instance.

However, go gently. A detox should be a nice rest for your body, rather than a deprivation or a sudden shock. So if you eat meat every day, cutting it out of your diet completely could be tough on your body. Reduce the amount you eat rather than completely stopping.

Don't look for a silver bullet; there isn't one. If you overdo things on the detox front, you will just be starving yourself. Detoxification has to happen naturally in the body on a continual basis. Your main job with a detox regime is to give your liver and gut the things they need to keep healthy, while removing other elements of your diet. When you get back to normal eating, your liver and gut should be stronger and healthier, and do a better job of daily detoxification.

ACTION POINTS

1. Choose a good couple of weeks to do a detox, when you're not under too much stress, or traveling.

2. Design your detox so that you're making a definite change from your normal diet, but not too severely. Find three or four foods or drinks mentioned in the detox chapter that you want to focus on, such as green tea, green vegetables, apples, and lemon juice. This means you've always got something appropriate in the pantry and you don't need to think too hard about what to eat.

3. Don't forget to keep your food diary during detox. Particularly, write down if you get any food cravings, and equally if they go away after a while.

4. Remember to keep well hydrated. You might actually want to track your liquid intake, a good way of seeing whether your normal regimen gives you enough water. Don't forget to do regular exercise while you're detoxing!

Chapter 7
HEAL AND NOURISH THE GUT

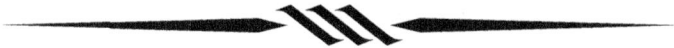

A s I mentioned before, I have IBS and I have to be careful what I eat; I don't want to trigger another big flare-up. But one of my friends is quite the opposite. I used to tell her she had a stomach made of iron – she could eat anything, and she never had any problems. She travelled around the world for six months before she went to college, eating street food, and she never got a single bug.

Then she had a small operation. The wound got infected, and she was given antibiotics to stop the infection. And suddenly, she was always getting ill; her digestion was delicate all of a sudden, and she couldn't work out why.

We now know that antibiotics can really take it out on your GI tract; they kill loads of microorganisms, and your whole gut microbiome suffers. That's what had happened to my friend. Fortunately, she ended up finding out about probiotics, and managed to kick-start her intestinal flora again.

But that experience with antibiotics, as well as a modern diet, which doesn't help the growth of the right microorganisms, is why many of us have digestive problems. So, we often need to take action to heal our digestive system, and then nurture and care for it till it's properly re-established.

Fermented foods

First of all, let's think about superfoods for probiotics – foods that are particularly rich in microorganisms. That means, in many cases, fermented foods. If you like Korean food, you're in luck – kimchi, the fermented cabbage which is a side dish for virtually every Korean meal, is a really good food in this regard. Different brands come with different amounts of chili, so you may want to try a few before you find just the right mix. Alternatively, learn to make it yourself; it's not that difficult, and if it's made at home, you know there are no added preservatives.

Sauerkraut is the northern European version of kimchi – fermented cabbage, but without the chili. It's often eaten as part of a rich meal with four or five different kinds of pork, but it's far more flexible than its traditional usage suggests. It can be used as a side dish, or baked with apples and sultanas for a little sweetness, used in soups or casseroles, or with potato to make latkes.

Gherkin pickles, if they have been properly pickled, are very tasty, go with any number of different meals, and are actually a great snack if you feel tempted outside of mealtimes. You may need to look around to find a good local provider, as some supermarket gherkins are just put in a weak sugar and vinegar solution, which won't give you any probiotic benefits, even though the gherkins will still be just as crunchy. 'Kosher dill pickles' are usually brined; labels that mention the words 'fermented,' 'unpasteurized,' or 'probiotic' indicate real pickles, whereas if vinegar is listed among the ingredients, you can assume the pickles aren't 'real.'

A fermented drink you could consider is kombucha. It starts off as black tea, and a bacteria/yeast colony nicknamed a SCOBY is used to ferment it. It's well known in China and Japan, and has become increasingly popular in the West. However, a number of extreme claims have been made for its health-giving properties, such as that it can cure AIDS, arthritis, anorexia, and cancer. Scientists have not found any truth in these claims and it's possible that kombucha could have adverse effects on your liver or kidneys, so be careful if you are adding it to your diet. Note that the fermentation can also result in kombucha containing alcohol.

If you're making your own kombucha, be careful that you keep your preparation clean; brew it in a glass, not metal container, and don't drink too much.

Natto is a Japanese food made from fermented soybeans. It's often eaten with rice, but it's an acquired taste – it's slippery and slimy, and smells of ammonia or old cheese. You may be able to guess that I'm not a fan, but others (including most of the population of Japan) are. It contains plenty of fiber and protein as well as probiotics and vitamin K2, and is a thoroughly healthy dish.

Miso, another Japanese fermented food, is probably more approachable for most of us than natto. Rice, barley, or soybean is fermented with the koji fungus for anything from days to years until it makes a smooth paste. There is rich, dark brown miso, fudge-colored miso, and even 'white' miso, which is more delicately flavored.

An Indonesian way of fermenting soybeans is tempeh, but instead of a paste, it's a kind of dough-like block. You can use it just like tofu, as a meat substitute. It absorbs other flavors quickly, so you can marinate it for half an hour in garlic and soy sauce, for instance, and it will taste garlicky and salty. You can eat it raw, too. And it freezes well, so if it's a bit difficult for you to get, you can buy in bulk and freeze what you don't need right now. Rich in probiotics, tempeh is also thought to reduce cholesterol, and provides plenty of calcium for your bones as well as lots of protein.

If you've visited Ukraine or Eastern Europe, you may know kvass, a rich and refreshing dark brown drink made by fermenting rye or barley, stale bread, or sometimes beets, with lactobacillus. It tastes not unlike a slightly soured dark beer - but it usually contains about 1% alcohol, so it's okay to drink a good sized glass of it and you won't fall over (don't leave it to ferment too long, though, or it will get stronger – it's best drunk fresh). You can make it yourself using baker's yeast, brewer's yeast or sourdough starter.

For some of these foods, you may need to look in a health food store rather than the supermarket. You may also want to ensure that pickles are actually fermented; some store-bought sauerkraut, for instance, hasn't been fermented but just quickly pickled, and that doesn't create the microorganisms you'd expect in a fermented food.

FERMENTED FOOD AND DRINK

- Kimchi
- Sauerkraut
- Gherkin pickles
- Kombucha
- Natto
- Miso
- Tempeh
- Kvass

Prebiotics, postbiotics and probiotics

Look at pre-, pro- and postbiotic supplements. While eating a good diet is the best and most effective way of keeping your gut healthy, supplements can make a big difference in a relatively short while, and can keep your gut microbiota on track. Don't worry if you're on the pill, by the way; probiotics and prebiotics won't affect the effectiveness of your contraception. They don't affect hormone levels in the body. And they won't interfere with other medications, either. In fact, if you're taking the pill, you might know that it can sometimes disrupt the gut microbiome, so taking probiotics can help you stay healthy.

Terminology can be confusing, so let's summarize here what each kind of supplement can do for you.

- Prebiotics are supplements that prepare the environment for your gut microbiota and give them the food they need.

- Probiotics are actual live bacteria and other microorganisms. By taking a supplement, you are creating fresh colonies of these beneficial microorganisms that can help keep your gut healthy.

- Postbiotics are generally produced by your gut microbiome and help your body regulate itself. However, if you have gut health issues, you might need to supplement these products, because your gut isn't producing enough of them.

We also looked earlier at how eating the right foods can help to reduce inflammation. The pill can increase levels of inflammation in the body, leading to period pain and PMS, aches and pains and creaky joints. So you're supporting your body against inflammation, too, if your diet supports a healthy gut, or if you take a probiotic supplement.

Probiotics

Brine-cured olives are full of probiotics, but you have to be careful to find a good brand, preferably organic. If they contain sodium benzoate as an additive, you've undone all the health benefits (yes, you have got to get used to scrutinizing the small print on food labels if you want to look after your digestive system!).

I already mentioned kefir in the last chapter. If you can make your own kefir, you've got access to some really powerful and diverse probiotics that should help you rebalance your gut microbiome. Coconut milk kefir isn't as high in probiotics as milk kefir, but it's still good for you.

I make a cup of miso soup some days for lunch; it's as easy as making tea! Just boil some water, put a teaspoonful of miso in a mug, pour the water over, and stir till it's dissolved into the water. It's surprisingly filling, which makes it a great ally if you're trying to lose weight! And it comes with a big load of probiotics to help your gut microbiome.

Yogurt is one of the easiest probiotic foods to acquire and you can use it in just about anything. Use it as a salad dressing or a topping for baked potato, add fruit to it, make frozen yogurt in summer, add it to sauces, eat it on rice or stir it into soup. But watch out – you want live yogurt, not pasteurized. And don't buy sweetened or flavored yogurt, which often has additional ingredients you don't want, such as artificial sweeteners and flavorings.

If you live near a farmers' market or a whole food shop where you can find local yogurt from grass-fed cows' or goats' milk, you'll be getting the best probiotic addition to your diet. If you're lactose intolerant, try to find coconut-milk yogurt – though again, check that it has live cultures.

Live buttermilk has some of the same properties as yogurt. It's the milk that's left over after churning butter – you may see it labeled as 'traditional.' It has less lactose than regular milk, which can help you if you have a mild lactose intolerance, and contains calcium. Make sure you buy buttermilk with active, live cultures. Buttermilk also has other benefits: it's full of vitamin B, can reduce acidity if you've eaten spicy or oily foods, and delivers a protein boost, too. It can help lower your cholesterol levels, reduce blood pressure, and even help with weight loss, because drinking buttermilk will make you feel full without consuming large amounts of calories.

Kvass has a wide range of probiotics but also delivers potassium, and vitamins A and C. Some people say it's an acquired taste, but I seem to have acquired it – which I haven't with kombucha!

Raw cheeses and raw milk have good probiotic content, but some places don't allow milk to be sold unpasteurized. If you can get raw milk locally, do. Raw cheeses will give you a choice of microorganisms – *thermophillus*, *bulgaricus*, *acidophilus*, and *bifidus*, to name just a few.

Apple cider vinegar is another good source of probiotics, and it's easy to use in your salad dressings, or to drink it, mixed with water and honey. Though fresh apples aren't fermented, they are also a good source of probiotics.

By the way, if you want to eat these foods for probiotics, make sure they haven't been pasteurized. That kills all the microorganisms.

KEFIR

Kefir is similar to, but a little thinner than, yogurt. You take cow or goat milk, and add kefir grains. These are actually small colonies of yeast and lactic acid bacteria that form a starter culture, and they work to ferment the milk over about twenty-four hours. They ferment all the sugars in the milk so that it turns into kefir, and you can then take the grains out of the liquid to reuse them.

Kefir is low in fat but high in certain nutrients. One cup gives you a quarter of your daily calcium needs, and a fifth of your daily phosphorous requirement, plus vitamin K2, which is also important to keeping your bones strong and healthy. It also contains plenty of vitamins B12, B2, and D, plus even more probiotics than yogurt, which can help reboot your digestive system during a detox. It includes a unique lactobacillus, *Lactobacillus kefiri*, which can protect you against *salmonella* and *E.coli*, and has anti-inflammatory effects.

Kefir is considerably lower in lactose than milk, so if you have a slight lactose intolerance, it may be a good alternative to full-lactose dairy. In fact, you can make non-dairy kefir using coconut milk or fruit juice, but because the chemistry will be different, you might not get all the benefits mentioned above. In particular, water-based kefir won't contain the protein and calcium content that's found in milk kefir. You'll also need to find a different type of kefir from the type used to make milk kefir. Look online for 'water kefir.'

To make kefir, get some kefir grains from a whole food shop or supermarket, and put them in a glass jar or bowl. Cover them with milk, cover the container and leave it at room temperature (22-25 C, 70-77 F) for at least twenty-four hours. You can then strain the kefir with a normal sieve. Put the liquid in the fridge and use the grains to start your next batch.

Make sure to buy kefir grains, sometimes sold as 'kefir starter kit.' Kefir sold in most supermarkets as a drink has been pasteurized, so it won't ferment and you will just end up with sour milk.

Prebiotics

Now let's look at prebiotics. Probiotics will help repopulate your gut microbiome; prebiotics, on the other hand, give the microorganisms in your gut something to work on. If you eat loads of probiotics but no prebiotics, it's like trying to drive fast with no petrol in the tank, or putting fish in your pond but not feeding them.

If you've read this far, it's not going to come as a surprise that some of the best prebiotics sources are leafy greens. They pack a lot of goodness in the form of vitamins B, C, and K, as well as plenty of minerals. Try just mixing a handful of leaves into any soups, stews, or curries, nibble at bit of arugula at the start of a meal, or put a bit of basil or cilantro in your smoothies. If you make a habit of putting a few leaves in every meal, you're going to find it much easier to make sure you have enough greens in your diet.

Although leeks aren't usually included under the heading of leafy greens, in this case, they probably should be. They contain inulin, also found in bananas and asparagus; it's a prebiotic that will really help beneficial bacteria in your GI tract.

Oats are another good source of prebiotics. In fact, I'd say that if you go out and grab yourself a packet of good oats (not the 'instant porridge' kind), that's probably the easiest way to build prebiotics into your diet.

To make overnight oats, stir milk, water, a plant-based milk or yogurt into the oats before you go to bed, and they'll be ready to eat in the morning – nicely softened up and with the beta-glucan prebiotics ready for your gut microorganisms to work on. Add fruit for a really healthy breakfast (I add blueberries, cinnamon, flax and hemp seed to my oats and eat them with almond milk).

Apples contain pectin, which you've heard of if you've ever tried to make jam – it's the agent that makes the jam 'set.' Pectin is also a great prebiotic. So apples – fresh, stewed, or baked - are another good source of prebiotics. Citrus fruits also include pectin.

Ginger contains prebiotics and can help digestion. Folk medicine used it to stop flatulence, and using ginger in your stir-fries can help your digestion. Or you can drink ginger tea, which can also help with digestion and I find is a great help if I'm feeling a bit under the weather; it always picks me up and helps with nausea too.

Postbiotics

Postbiotics exist too, though you don't hear so much about them as about pre- and probiotics. Postbiotics are produced by microorganisms when they process nutrients; if your gut is doing its job properly, it will produce such things as butyric acid and acetic acid. Postbiotics are really useful in helping keep your body healthy, but if you don't produce enough of them, or if you are ill, taking postbiotic supplements can help get you back in balance. For instance, postbiotics have been shown to help with rhinitis and eczema, and with colic in babies, as well as with IBS.

Tongue scraping

Add a tongue scrape to your dental regime. You can buy a dedicated tool, or just use the tongue cleaner on the back of your toothbrush (using the brush itself is not really effective). Be very gentle; brush your teeth first, then scrape from the back of your tongue towards your teeth. Your aim is to remove dead cells from the top of the tongue. By doing so, you can improve your sense of taste, and get rid of bad breath. There are also a few nasty bacteria that tend to hang around in your mouth, like *Mutans streptococci*, and this will help to deter them.

If you gag, you just started too far back, so try again from further forwards. Then wash your mouth out with water a few times and don't forget to wash your scraper properly.

How to keep on the right track

'Healthy eating' always sounds so boring. I'm sure many of us have memories from childhood of being forced to eat things we found unpalatable, and being told it was good for us. Maybe we have friends whose entire diet seems to be based around wheatgrass smoothies. So it can be difficult to keep on the right track, particularly when the internet, the TV, and the papers are all full of ads for all those foods you're trying to avoid. So here are a few tips for staying the course.

First, think of your gut-healthy diet as a chance to try food you've never had. Travel the world with your diet: try Japanese seaweed-wrapped rice balls... try fish or veg that you never ate before. Grab a cookbook and learn how to cook Indian, Thai, or Korean style – there are plenty of good books for beginners – or learn how to make your own pickles.

Share food with other people. If you have friends who want to eat healthily and try new dishes, why don't you take it in turns to cook for each other at the weekends? And talk about food, too – if you shop at a farmer's market or in a minority-owned shop and you don't know what to do with a particular vegetable or fruit, ask! I've had some great conversations in little stores where people told me how to cook yam, pak choi, and plantain (unripe banana), and often, other customers joined in with their own advice and recipes.

Make what you eat interesting. You don't have to spend a trillion hours at the stove to do this; just make a few intelligent tweaks. Chicken breast can be spiced up so easily with a cayenne-based rub, mustard crust, lemon slices on top, feta cheese stuffing, lime juice marinade, honey-vinegar sauce, or jerk seasoning. Add some mango salsa, wilted spinach, arugula, or bake some tomatoes alongside the chicken to add a bit more variety.

Make salsa and sauce you can freeze for later. Homemade tomato sauce is so much better than store bought – you can add chilis for a bit of heat, too. Make enough for four or five batches at a time and you can make any dish more interesting by just microwaving up that sauce.

Learn to cook 'en papilotte,' in little folded baking paper packets. You can put the whole meal in one package and bake or steam it, which is a healthy way to cook, and keeps all the flavor inside. For instance, put a piece of salmon with a few slices of lemon, shredded carrots, sliced courgette, chopped leeks or sliced fennel, wrap it up properly and bake for about twenty minutes. The unwrapping, of course, is the best part!

Mix up the colors for visual appeal. Serve broccoli and red cabbage, for instance, or avocado and tomatoes. Blanch green vegetables first if you are going to cook them – put them in boiling water for a couple of minutes, then drain quickly and refresh with running cold water; this keeps their color bright and green. I also roast mine.

Supplements

My whole approach in this book has been to find natural ways to stimulate your gut microbiome and look after your gut health. But for some of us, supplements are a useful way to get started, and that's particularly the case if you've been in hospital, or on antibiotics, which can be really disruptive to your GI tract.

As we know, probiotic supplements provide the actual microorganisms that inhabit your gut. Prebiotics provide the types of carbs or fiber that beneficial bacteria in your gut can eat. Many supplements will contain both, mixed together. To choose the right supplements, look for a diversity of different bacteria. Taking a supplement is very low risk, unless you have a chronic disease, in which case you should talk to your doctor first.

L-glutamine is currently trendy, and can be useful; this too is low risk. There is some research showing it can be useful in managing IBS, as it can boost immune cell activity in the gut. It may be particularly useful if you're following a low-FODMAP diet, as many of the foods that such diets exclude are good sources of glutamine. However, it's not a magic bullet. Find out the real reason for your gut problems before you consider taking it.

Collagen is usually thought of as beneficial to the skin, keeping it elastic. But it's also good for the gut, as it includes glycine, proline and glutamine, three amino acids which can help keep the lining of your GI tract in good shape. Our bodies produce collagen, but we produce less of it as we age, so taking a supplement is one way of putting it back into your system. You could eat lots of bone marrow, bone broth, and gelatin, or you could take collagen peptide supplements. These won't be suitable for vegetarians, though, as they're either made of marine collagen from fish or bovine collagen from cow hide.

A vegetarian-friendly way of addressing collagen deficiency is to support your own body's collagen production by making sure you have plenty of glycine. You can get this from sesame, pumpkin and sunflower seeds, spirulina, nori and other seaweeds, watercress, spinach, and beans.

Licorice root, often used as a sweetener, also contains glycyrrhizin, which can help to heal stomach ulcers by increasing mucus production in the stomach. But don't take it if you are (or are trying to get) pregnant – licorice can lead to fetal development problems, a risk not worth taking.

While you might decide that changing your diet has brought enough benefits and you don't need supplements, they can nonetheless be a good way of supporting long-term gut health as well as kick-starting your gut microbiome. But you do need to choose your supplements carefully.

In the next chapter, we'll look at how to keep going in the long term. We all know how easy it is to go on a diet and lose a few pounds, and how difficult it is to keep it off, and the same is true of your gut health.

ACTION POINTS

1. Go through the chapter and write down all the foods mentioned that you really like eating, and all the foods you haven't tried. This is your recipe book for your gut-healthy diet!

2. Have a go at making your own kefir. You never know, you may be a natural.

3. Find a healthy diet/gut buddy and agree to take it in turns at weekends to cook healthy meals. Be adventurous.

Chapter 8
RETAINING GOOD LONG-TERM GUT HEALTH THROUGH DIET

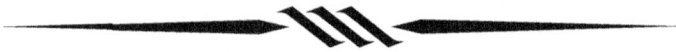

————————)))) ————————

E ating a gut-friendly diet is often easy – as long as you think it will be over soon – but staying faithful to your new good habits in the long term can be difficult. You need some good strategies to see when you're going wrong and to help you get back on track, and that's what this chapter should provide.

One thing that really helps is to keep trying new foods. If you're bored of green leafy vegetables, try another food that delivers the same bunch of nutrients and probiotics. Try quinoa, tofu, beansprouts, persimmons, mango, plantain, physalis, or Jerusalem artichokes. Look for new recipes if you feel you're getting in a rut, or find a new spice you haven't tried before.

Never had oysters? Sushi? Seaweed? Buckwheat noodles? A really stinky cheese? It's time to try!

Get to recognise that feeling of being stuck in a rut, before you start heading for the comfort food. Sometimes, it can be a good idea to say "Okay, let's eat out," but pick a cuisine you don't know very well, or dishes you haven't eaten before, and let that give you inspiration.

I'm always shocked when I see people throwing pumpkins away after Halloween. I feel like shouting "Hey! Don't you know you can eat that?"

If you have children, you'll be teaching them by example that it's worth trying new things, and you'll like some but maybe not others. They'll grow up feeling happy to test whatever the world of food has to offer. It doesn't mean they will like everything, but it *does* mean they're unlikely to be picky eaters.

We so easily get into habits – always using spaghetti when there are so many other types of pasta you could use, for instance. So shake things up time to time, to keep your appetite fresh.

Cravings are something we all have to deal with occasionally. If you just try to suppress the craving, you're going to be thinking about the thing you crave all the time – it's like that game where you have to *not* think about unicorns, or elephants, or whatever.

Certain foods are designed for us to crave – pretzels, candies, junk food, cookies. They have high fat and high sugar, plus extra-strong flavorings to knock our taste buds out. We start wanting everything to taste really salty, really sugary, really fatty. We lose our palates for delicate flavors.

So to resist these cravings, you need a reset. You need to start appreciating how tasty fruit and veg can be without added sugar. That can mean getting extra picky about fruit being properly ripe, and about vegetables being cooked just right, but it's worth it. Add umami, a great savory flavor that comes from mushrooms, miso paste, soy sauce or fish sauce, instead of salt.

You can really get used to it. After about a year of healthy eating, I let myself have a McDonald's and a vanilla milkshake. I couldn't get over how weird it tasted compared to my regular diet!

Make the healthy option the easy one. Often, salty, fatty and sugary snacks are the easiest to reach for when you are peckish. Have plenty of healthy foods you can eat just as they are for an easy snack – dates, chopped carrots, dried apricots, fresh grapes, sunflower seeds. I like to nibble on houmous and rice cakes.

Put your healthy options at the front of the fridge and out on the counter. Put fruit in a bowl on the table. If you have less healthy food at home, put it where it's more difficult to reach. If you have a healthy plan for the sneaky little hunger that arrives mid-morning or in the late afternoon, you're leaving cravings no way in the door.

So every morning, I like to arrange my snacking plan. "If I'm hungry between lunch and dinner ... I'm going to eat some raspberries." Or "If I'm hungry before I go to bed ... I'm going to have a half a cup of miso soup." So then I know exactly what I'm going to do; I won't just go into the kitchen and look for something to eat. And I won't suddenly be craving cookies, because cookies aren't an option; the raspberries are already pre-planned.

Cutting out processed foods completely, if you can, is great. It will make you feel so much better. You'll be cutting out 'empty' calories (calories with minimal nutrients), excessive salt and sugar, and cheap oils with too much saturated fat and not enough omega-3. You'll also cut out a load of preservatives, colorings and flavorings.

Eating out

But sometimes you want to eat out. You may be fortunate enough to know local restaurants or cafes where food is prepared freshly from minimally processed foods. But without asking the chef for the entire written recipe, how do you pick the healthiest option? Remember, if you want a healthy GI tract, you want to make sure you eat as healthily as possible, so make mindful choices.

MINDFUL CHOICES

- Less usual grains like amaranth, buckwheat, sorghum, quinoa and wild rice are practically never processed, so they'll be wholegrain; as will bulgur wheat and brown rice. Otherwise, look on the label for 'wholegrain,' 'whole wheat' and so on.

- Vegetable salads are usually minimally processed, but beware of dressings! If they come just with vinaigrette or with the dressing provided on the side, you'll minimise the chances of getting a load of fat, sugar, salt and flavorings.

- Dishes such as curries, stews, and pies, are more likely to have been made with processed ingredients than, say, a poached chicken breast or a minute steak.

- A restaurant which makes the main dishes itself may still buy in the desserts, which means they may use a lot of processed fats and other ingredients. Skipping dessert is often sensible.

- Restaurants with vegan and vegetarian choices will usually have put a lot of thought into healthy ingredients, and probably use organic sources of supply.

- Avoid fried foods which could be cooked in processed fats. Watch out for words like 'crispy,' 'scalloped,' and 'breaded.'

- 'Creamy' is another giveaway word! It may mean cream, or it may mean hydrogenated vegetable fat; either way, it's not going to be healthy.

- Restaurants which boast that they use local sources for their dishes often use fewer processed ingredients, too.

- Fish, unless buttered or fried, is often one of the healthiest dishes.

- Ask for water with your meal; a slice of lime or lemon can make it more palatable.

You can always ask for the manager or chef to help you choose. Explain that you're trying to stay healthy, and your diet means you have to be a little careful. Explain exactly what you want to avoid, and ask for their help in choosing the best dish. A friendly approach will rarely offend, and you're also making life easier for others who are trying to make healthy choices. Or you could ask for a sauce or a particular ingredient to be missed out.

Healthy eating can be difficult if your friends all want to order the 'unhealthy' option. Sometimes, it's easier if you order first. You might also want to try ordering two appetizers rather than a starter and a main course, or ask the server to swap part of your meal for a healthier option, like having extra vegetables instead of French fries.

If the portions are huge, you could even ask for half your entree to be put in a doggy bag *before* it's served. That stops you feeling any psychological pressure to clear your plate, and gives you something to look forward to tomorrow.

To avoid snacking on the bread rolls or sticks, have a little nibble – some nuts or seeds, or an apple – before you go.

But don't forget, if you're eating out, to have some fun too! It's only your birthday or your wedding anniversary once a year, so let yourself off the leash a bit. Just remember to get back into healthy eating again afterwards. Don't try to starve the next day to make up for the treat; just get back into your regular healthy diet.

Long-term habits

The best diet is one you can stick to. If you're too ambitious, and change what you eat too drastically, you can end up feeling food cravings all the time, and you're not going to stay on the straight and narrow. If you try to eat food you don't actually like, just because it's healthy, you're going to be easily tempted to replace it by a less healthy alternative. This is one of the problems with fashionable fad diets: they lead to yo-yo behavior. You lose a bit of weight with the diet, come off the diet and put the weight back on, then go back on the diet to try to lose it again. And all that yo-yoing isn't very good for your body. It can actually wreak havoc on your gut microbiome. So when you're thinking about food for gut health, make sure you can live with your decisions. Go gently!

We talked about elimination diets earlier. Remember, those are simply a diagnostic tool for finding out if you have food intolerances, and they last just five or six weeks. They are definitely not proposed as a long-term diet regime. In fact, if a diet is too restrictive, it's usually a sign that it's not a good one. If you're only allowed to eat one kind of food, whether it's cabbage soup or potatoes, avocadoes or raw meat, your body is not going to benefit.

If you're always feeling hungry or thirsty, you need to adapt your eating plan. Drinking plenty of water (or herbal tea) will help (with the hunger as well as the thirst), and so will eating fiber-rich fruit and veg. You should feel well nourished, and energetic, else you're not doing it right.

Find a plan that fits your lifestyle. For instance, if you travel regularly for your work, you'll need to give yourself some flexibility or you could find yourself skipping meals because you can't find the right food. If you have children and your regime doesn't include stuff they'll find edible, you're going to end up cooking two dinners and two breakfasts, which is hard work.

It's the same with exercise: it needs to fit your lifestyle and be enjoyable. Every year, people join up at the gym as a New Year's resolution, and by February they've stopped going. Perhaps they don't like the atmosphere, or it's too far out of their way, or they don't have a good time slot for it, or they realize they really needed to get a bit fitter generally before they started trying to lift weights. You might be better joining in with a more social form of exercise, like zumba, dancing, five-a-side soccer, or Parkrun, or just getting up early for a walk or run round the block.

We've talked about how some foods are better than others for your gut. But it's an odd thing that in Western culture, we love to define some foods as 'good' and others as 'bad.' Plenty of diets have long lists of 'forbidden' food. If you really love a glass of chardonnay or a craft beer from time to time, then don't consider them forbidden. They're treats, and you can certainly have one from time to time (well, not when you're detoxing, perhaps). Chocolate? Fine, but spend money on a really good dark chocolate, rather than binge-eating Reese's Peanut Butter Cups (don't ask me how I know about binge-eating Reese's Peanut Butter Cups!).

In fact, the 80/20 rule isn't a bad one to apply to your food. I know it from my life in business, as very often, the 80/20 rule applies to which products make you the most profit, or which changes will bring about the greatest benefits, or focusing 80% of your time on your strengths and 20% on your weaknesses. So, you could eat gut-friendly foods 80% of the time, and the other 20% of the time, you can add something you enjoy but that doesn't fall into that list. Or you might say, "80% of the month I will eat what's recommended, and that leaves me a pocket of permissions to dine out with friends." As long as you're not totally splurging with that 20%, this can keep you motivated to have a healthy diet *most* of the time. I tend to be strict Monday to Friday and add a few treats in at weekend or on vacations.

Take things gently. Change is difficult. You don't have to change everything all at once. One thing you can do is to think what is the single most beneficial change you can make to your health through diet or exercise right now, and just do that. Try to make it a positive, not a negative. Saying "I will give up cookies" is less likely to succeed than "I will eat two fermented foods every day" or "I will have a homemade vegetable salad or soup for lunch." Or you could find the easiest thing to change, and change that. Just making yourself 'overnight oats' for breakfast, for instance, could get every day off to a great start.

Have plenty of variety in your diet. If you just eat your way through spinach and tomato salad every lunchtime, it may be healthy, but you're going to get bored. You might decide that you're going to try new dishes every weekend, when you have a bit more time to cook. You might make up a new spice blend to use as a spice rub on meat or chicken, or take ideas from traditional spice blends like North African ras el-hanout (cumin, ground ginger, turmeric, cinnamon, black pepper, coriander seed, cayenne pepper, nutmeg and cloves) or panch puran from Punjab (fenugreek, nigella, cumin, mustard and fennel seed).

Make your own lunchtime salads. If making your own hummus from chickpeas, for instance, you can add all kinds of flavors (lemon, cilantro, paprika), or you could make coleslaw and add grapefruit, or sunflower seeds, or a little Thai curry paste. The possibilities are endless! You can make your own cucumber and yogurt salad, or you can roast vegetables in the oven and keep them in the fridge for a few days as a great cold lunch. Add some olives and goat's cheese and you have a great variety to load your plate with.

Remember that food is your energy source. You have to get all the nutrients you need – carbs, fats and proteins, but also vitamins and minerals. Be conscious of what each food gives you, and also be certain about what you're eating; that means checking the label, buying fresh and buying local when you can.

Some quite simple tricks can make your life much easier.

FOOD HACKS

- Buy smaller plates! If you tend to overeat, a dainty plate can make you feel you're eating more, while you're actually eating less.

- Half your plate should be full of green and red – non-starchy veg like carrots, tomatoes, leafy greens, or courgette. They will fill you up and deliver a load of nutrients without too many calories.

- Eat morning oats? Always add some fruit!

- Shop after you've eaten. If you shop when you're hungry, you will buy higher-calorie foods and probably less healthy ones.

- Drink green tea or water with every meal.

- Have dry beans, pulses, quinoa, oats and rice at home so you always have something healthy in store. Frozen vegetables can also be good, but check the label – some stir-fry mixes have additional, less desirable ingredients; broccoli, spinach, and carrots are particularly useful frozen vegetables.

- Make up ice cubes with spinach, herbs like cilantro, and other vegetables. You can then just pop a couple of cubes into a soup or stew.

- Keep healthy snacks easily accessible. Have a fruit bowl on the dining table or even in your office.

- If you love coffee, have an espresso, not a full cream latte with extra caramel syrup. You're probably going to save about 250 calories making that switch!
- If you don't love cold salad, try a warm salad. This could be a regular lettuce and tomato salad but with four slices of warm goat's cheese added, or a wilted spinach salad just given enough time in the pan to warm it up. I add buckwheat pasta.
- Use a spiralizer to make veggie 'noodles' with zucchini or squash.
- Use mushrooms or chickpeas to add 'meatiness' to a dish. Dried mushrooms from an Asian supermarket can make a good last-minute addition.
- Add plant-based 'milks' to your diet. Cashew and coconut milk are rich and creamy; almond milk is refreshing.
- For exercise, keep small free weights on a table or shelf you need to go past a few times a day, and do ten or twenty repetitions every time you go past!

An easy way to keep eating healthier is to try to add more plant-based food to each meal (remember, plants have fiber, meat doesn't). Add soybean-based products like edamame (unripe soybeans, great for snacking on), tofu, tempeh, and miso. Mix chickpeas into a stew or soup; add nuts and seeds to your breakfast oats, salad dressings, or yogurt. Add a handful of salad leaves to anything (except perhaps desserts!). Most things you can cook with minced beef, you can cook with beans. Just by adding a little extra plant-based food to your meals, you're automatically reducing the amount of saturated fat you're eating.

Eating soy is good; eating the right kind of soy is better! As with other foods, you want to eat a minimally processed form of soybean. So sweetened soy milks and yogurts are not the ideal way to get your soy fix; nor is soy 'meat.' Instead, pick tofu, edamame, beansprouts, or fermented soy products like miso and tempeh.

If a local business offers direct-to-doorstep vegetable boxes from local producers, that's a great way to get more veg into your diet. It can also be quite fun finding recipes for some of the more unusual veg, plus you're supporting small business.

Mindful eating

Mindful eating can be a very powerful way to keep motivated and keep on track with new, healthy eating habits.

Slow down a bit. Eating fast can mean you don't give your body enough time to adjust, so you eat too much before your body has got round to telling you, "That's enough." Don't eat on the go, or in a hurry, or on the couch; sit down, slow down, let yourself feel your tummy getting full.

Tune into your body between and before meals. Are you really hungry? Do you just want a nibble? Are you feeling a bit dehydrated or light-headed? We often listen to our emotions rather than our bodies about food, leading to comfort eating, and that leads not just to eating too much, but to eating the wrong things. I often feel like reaching for the chocolate when feeling down but have learnt to control this. Feel your stomach growling, or other symptoms of hunger, and learn to recognize those signals. If your body isn't hungry, you know that your mind is using food as a distraction.

Mindful eating isn't about rules. It's about appreciation and consideration. Treat every mouthful as a gourmet experience. Think about where your food came from, and about how it was cooked, perhaps about the cooking tradition and where you learned to cook the dish. Experience the food when you put it in your mouth, then when you bite on it, then when you swallow it. Let yourself savor it for a moment before taking another mouthful. You are just experiencing the food, not being judgmental about whether you 'should' be eating it, coming to every mouthful as if for the first time.

ACTION STEPS

1. Work out what percentage of your diet consists of highly processed foods. Then think about ways to reduce your consumption of these foods.

2. Find new addictions. Instead of the salt/sugar mix of processed foods, find natural foods that you love. For me, strawberries, blueberries and raspberries are my 'fix,' and miso soup is my go-to easy-to-make food for when I'm tired and hungry.

3. A great way to start mindful eating is just to cook one vegetable and try to get all the flavor out of it. For instance, roast some asparagus spears with a tiny dab of butter; steam your broccoli instead of boiling it, and add a squeeze of lemon; bake cherry tomatoes till they split, then add a little balsamic vinegar. Focus on that vegetable and really taste it; savor the aromas and the texture as well.

4. If you enjoy eating out, find restaurants that serve healthy food, whether they are vegan, serve local, seasonal food, or simply serve great salads. When you're traveling, use the internet to find great places to eat that will suit your diet and your pocketbook.

5. Create your healthy store cupboard. Replace cup-a-soups with miso, pretzels and chips with seeds and nuts, and candy bars with dried fruit. Add the herbs and spices you particularly like.

Chapter 9
STRESS AND SELF-CARE

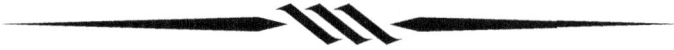

'Self-care' may make you think of saunas and candlelit baths, but it's not about pampering; it's about ensuring you are both physically and mentally healthy. It's something you need to do for yourself and for your family. To be healthy, you need to take care of yourself. You may need a doctor too, a midwife, or a therapist, but self-care is *your* part of the bargain. Self-care is really important if you have IBS, IBD or another gut condition, because of the brain/gut axis and the way stress affects your GI tract.

Don't neglect your mind. Depression and stress can make your body very sick, particularly when it comes to your gut. The first thing you need to learn is proper relaxation. Just five minutes of stepping away from stress, breathing deeply and relaxing your body can give you the groundedness and energy you need.

The connection between the mind and gut

An overactive mind means an overactive gut. The vagus nerve is central to the gut/brain axis; it's an immensely long nerve that runs all the way from the brain stem to the colon, and it controls your digestion, heart rate, and breathing. Reflexes such as sneezing, vomiting, and swallowing are all controlled by the vagus nerve; it also stimulates the unconscious contractions in your digestive tract which push food through the system.

Damage to the vagus nerve can bring about vomiting, acid reflux, bloating, and abdominal pain. It's also likely that the vagus nerve has something to do with depression. This is currently being researched, though the exact link is not known. It also affects inflammatory conditions such as rheumatoid arthritis.

Medics are now researching stimulation of the vagus nerve as an ancillary treatment for both gastric diseases and mental health problems such as depression and PTSD. Meditation and guided hypnotherapy have both been shown to be particularly beneficial when associated with electrical stimulation of the vagus nerve, either directly (through an implant) or through a device clipped to the ear.

Early-life trauma can change the microbiome, and in many cases this is linked to a susceptibility to depression. It is possible that deep breathing, as practised in pranayama and other meditations, can get the vagus nerve to trigger a relaxation response that can reduce heart rate and blood pressure, and that can help alleviate depression. It may also reduce symptoms associated with chronic pain.

Managing stress

Stress isn't bad – we need a bit of it – but being stressed *all* the time isn't healthy. It can let feelings of low self-esteem, depression, and anxiety overwhelm you; you may feel you just can't cope. Stress can also drive excessive drinking, overeating, aggression, and fatigue.

Yes, it's annoying when people say "just relax." You have to learn *how* to relax, and that can take time. To start with, you could schedule five minutes every morning and afternoon to use a basic relaxation technique.

BASIC RELAXATION TECHNIQUES

- Sit or lie down so you are comfortable.
- Focus on breathing slowly and deeply.
- Tighten and then relax each muscle in your body, starting from your head and neck and working downwards.
- Imagine a relaxing place, perhaps the seashore or a forest.
- Meditate (if you have learned how to do it).
- Walk mindfully.
- Watch the clouds mindfully.

At home, have a hot bath or listen to some good music. Some people even play music as a way to relax – I have a friend who plays flute for ten minutes every morning, just improvising and going with the flow.

More generally, find activities where you can get 'in the flow' and find self-fulfilment as well as relaxation. You might do calligraphy, paint, or throw pottery on the wheel. You might spend a few minutes every day on your balcony garden. You may have one or two friends in whose company you can really relax; schedule a cup of coffee with them every so often.

Make sure your friends and family know you need some downtime on your own. It's so easy to get drawn into commitments, and women are particularly likely to be called on for everything from grandchild-sitting to caring for the elderly, making food for get-togethers, doing the school run, and emergency cat-feeding or dog-walking duties.

Sometimes, though, if you have kids, you can relax by teaching *them* how to relax. Have 'silly time' together, thinking of the silliest things you could do, or singing a silly song; have some hugs, or some still time together, or take a walk with them. Make sure that they know it's a special time, though – and that you need it as much as they do!

Aromatherapy

I said self-care wasn't about pampering yourself, but with aromatherapy it can come quite close. Aromatherapy uses essential oils extracted from plants. It takes 200lb of lavender to make just 1lb of lavender oil, so they really pack a punch (and can also be quite expensive).

There's no real scientific evidence for how aromatherapy works; the oils *may* have an effect through stimulating your limbic system, which plays a role in your emotions. Or perhaps we just like pretty smells and they make us feel happy. But it's certain that a lot of people find these scents can help them relax and improve their sleep.

To use aromatherapy oils, you can use an infuser, or put a few drops on your pillow before you go to bed; you can mix them with massage oil and rub them into your skin; you can use a spritzer, or put them in your bath water. Just don't try to ingest them (also, keep them away from children under six).

Start with just two or three scents from this list:

- Lavender – decreases anxiety and improves sleep.
- Sweet orange, bergamot – increases energy and improves your mood.
- Rosemary – for mental alertness.
- Chamomile – for deep sleep.
- Sandalwood – reduces anxiety.
- Clary sage – reduces stress.
- Jasmine, lemon – good to lift your mood and avoid depression.

Herbs and herbal supplements

You might also use herbs and herbal supplements to look after yourself. Be careful that you know exactly what you're taking; some herbs have been found to have undesirable effects, for instance, kava impacts the liver. Even chamomile, which is an almost problem-free herb, can increase the risk of bleeding if you are taking blood-thinning drugs.

Lavender and lemon balm are usually well tolerated and can help reduce stress and anxiety. Use lavender in lavender bags, or in an infusion; lemon balm is best infused for a lightly lemon-scented drink.

Ashwagandha ('Indian ginseng') is used in ayurvedic medicine, and appears to help with stress, according to two studies of small groups of patients. It's usually taken as a capsule. However, it can affect blood sugar levels, so if you are diabetic, you should avoid it.

Passionflower is available in liquid tincture, or as tablets, and it can reduce anxiety. It's often recommended before surgery.

CBD is still rather controversial, but medical use of cannabis derivatives has increased over recent years. CBD can be *extracted* from cannabis or hemp, but it won't make you high, or give you the munchies. It *can* help to calm your nerves and relieve pain, and it's available as tablet, liquid extract or cream. It has also been suggested that it can reduce inflammation and pain from arthritis.

Taken in excess, CBD can make you irritable or nauseous, and it might affect the liver. Since it's not FDA regulated, the dose may not be exactly as stated on the label, so choose a reputable supplier. Also, do discuss the decision to take it with your doctor, in case you are taking a medication that could clash with it.

Art and creativity

Another part of self-care is looking after your own creativity and energy. Art and music should be a part of everyone's life. Find what you enjoy – strumming guitar, painting with watercolors, messy pottery, writing, collage, quilt-making. You don't have to try to be Shakespeare or Michelangelo; just enjoy the process of creating. Music, in particular, is a really good way of helping to manage emotions. That's one reason that occupational therapy departments exist in many hospitals.

YouTube is always a good source of ideas, and a lot of museums have virtual visits online.

RECREATING ART

During the pandemic, the Getty Museum challenged people to recreate famous works of art using the items they happened to have in the house. This inspired Peter Braithwaite, a British operatic baritone, who was unable to work as the opera houses were closed. Instead, he devoted himself to researching and recreating portraits of black people through history, using his acting flair to bring them to life. He has now published the results in a book, *Rediscovering Black Portraiture*.

Other people let their dogs, cats, and children star in recreations from the Botticelli Venus through Van Gogh all the way to David Hockney's famous *Paddling Pool (A Smaller Splash)*. Why not take up the challenge yourself to have some dressing-up fun, or create your own modern versions of classic paintings?

You could do a Zoom calligraphy get-together, or bring friends together for an afternoon of baking sourdough or writing haiku. If you have musical friends, you could make a band; if you have very different instruments and musical styles, part of the challenge will be finding a way to make them all work together. Or you could incorporate music into your life by listening to something new every day, or getting to know a new style (reggae? northern soul? Gregorian chants?). You could join an orchestra or a choir, or you could simply sing in the shower.

A friend has taken things a stage further with YouTube videos which have a scrolling score at the same time as the music plays – she find it soothing and it's really helped her to learn to read music. Sometimes she'll spend a few days following first one instrument in a string quartet, and then another, to see different facets of the music.

Coloring books are not just for kids any more; they're big sellers to adults.

And coloring does actually help you relax; in fact, it can have benefits similar to meditation. Use it as a pre-bedtime ritual, or as a way to unwind when you get home. It really takes your attention away from yourself and stressful thoughts, and if you tend to be perfectionist and judgmental about your own paintings, coloring has much lower stakes.

You might want to get involved in journaling. Using a gratitude journal lets you refocus on your day, getting away from the moment-to-moment stress and reflecting on what really mattered to you in each day. It's a way to clear your mind, 'putting the day to bed,' as it were. Or you can doodle (Zentangle can be addictive), or illustrate your day with pictures in the journal. Some people meditate before or after journaling, while others get energized first with some shakes and stretches.

Journaling can also help you to do meditation or yoga – or any other practice – in a more structured way. You can answer questions such as: "What was your intention for the practice?," "How was your breathing?," "How was your energy level?," "Did you find it difficult staying focused?," "How would you describe your practise today?," or "What is your next goal?" This can be really powerful when you look back and see how far you have come.

Exploring creativity with others can also really free your spirit and support your wellbeing. There's a concept of 'flow' that says when we 'go with the flow,' we are in our element, unaware of time, unstressed, calm and happy. Painting or even helping build a barn can help you to get there. Something that you find totally absorbing, that you can lose yourself in, helps to tap into this state of flow.

Having hobbies

We talked a little above about doing something creative. But your hobbies don't necessarily need to be creative. You might go walking, join a book club, or play soccer. Hobbies are great for bringing meaning to your life.

If you feel you're getting in a rut, try something new. Read a poem, visit an art gallery, take a martial arts class, learn a new skill, watch a film you've heard a lot about but never seen, travel somewhere you've not been before. Or revisit an old interest – maybe you gave it up when you moved and there wasn't a group in your new city; maybe you didn't have time when your children were small. Whatever the reason, pick it up and see if you get pulled into it again.

Meditation and mindfulness

Meditation is a great way to wipe away stress and achieve wellbeing, and you only need a few minutes to do it, though some people can sit in meditation for hours. You can do it anywhere: on the bus, walking, in the dentist's waiting room, in the restaurant, in your car, at your desk. It's not necessary to believe in any particular spiritual tradition to have a practice of mindfulness or meditation; it's just about being quiet and listening to your mind's internal conversation without getting caught up in it.

Meditation teachers often talk about 'monkey mind' – the way our minds jump about from one thing to another. Meditation is meant to quieten your mind. If a thought pops into your head, you recognize it, and then leave it aside. So instead of your thoughts going "Mom's coming on Sunday... oh goodness, I need to clean the house, get the kids on their best behavior, order a turkey, get the guest bedroom ready... what did I do with the quilt for the bed? ..." you will just go: "Mom's coming on Sunday. Uh-huh, that's right, she's coming Sunday. OK, breathe...."

You just notice that your mind is jumping about, but you don't let it go off anywhere. In meditation, you just say to yourself, "Oh, my mind is worrying." You accept the fact that it's worrying, and then you let the worry go. Once you get the knack, it's a really amazing thing to be able to do that; it takes so much stress out of life.

There are different kinds of meditation. You can do a guided meditation. You can do pranayama, breath meditation. You might use a mantra; many Buddhists use 'Om mani padme hum,' ('Hail the jewel in the lotus,' but 'Om' is also said to be the primeval sound which created the world; some Tibetans use 'Om ah hum') while some Christians use the Maranatha ('Come, my Lord') mantra. In some schools, gurus give their pupils an individual mantra. But you don't need to be religious to meditate; 'supercalifragilisticexpialidocious' would work just fine! Using a repeated sound like a gong or singing bowl can also help you focus through sound.

Mindfulness meditation involves living fully in the moment. For instance, if you take a walk, but you are listening to the birds, to your footsteps, feeling the wind on your face, being fully aware of everything around you instead of having various thoughts running through your mind, that's a walking mindfulness meditation. Or you could use qi gong, tai chi or yoga as a way of meditating on your breath and on your body's energy flows.

Some people find it difficult to get started with meditation. Start with just a few minutes, and work up to longer periods of meditation. Try to stick to a couple of regular times, such as just before breakfast, or before going to bed. If you create a small altar or meditation sanctuary, that can help; you might always have a fresh flower in a vase, or have a silky, comfortable cushion, or a photo of clouds that can help your mind calm down when you look at it. You might even have a spot in your garden where you meditate.

Celebrate small achievements. If you meditate three days in a row, give yourself a present, whether that's just a pat on the back, or a ticket to a concert, or a box of sushi for lunch. Don't beat yourself up if you miss your meditation one day; just remember to do it tomorrow.

Deep breathing will help you manage stress, whether or not you pair it with meditation. If you look at a baby, or someone sleeping really peacefully, you'll see how they breathe really deeply, quite naturally. They don't move their shoulders, and when they inhale, they fill their entire abdomen up with air. You should be breathing from deep in your belly, not just from your chest. Put a hand on your belly and a hand on the small of your back and you'll be able to feel if you are breathing deeply enough – both hands ought to move.

As we grow up, we tend to lose our deep breathing, and instead, we breathe shallowly most of the time. You'll feel when you start breathing more deeply that you're accessing areas you're not used to: you may feel your ribs and even your back expanding. Don't forget to breathe all the way out – holding your breath is the worst thing you can do.

When you get good at this, you can visualize yourself taking in goodness out of the air as you breathe in, and getting rid of negative vibes, stress, aches and pains as you breathe out. And every so often, it's good to breathe out really hard – just let it all go, whoosh! That can be incredibly relaxing and get rid of a lot of tension in one go.

A deep breath or two can be a quick way to calm down if things are getting the better of you. Admit to yourself that you're getting stressed or angry – recognize the feeling – and then just breathe, concentrating on the feeling of those nice, deep breaths. You might find a mantra that works for you in these situations. I sometimes channel Scarlett O'Hara from 'Gone with the Wind,' and say "Tomorrow is another day."

Other people I know have a talisman that makes them feel grounded. One friend has a pebble with a hole in it that she found on the beach; just feeling it helps her feel more calm and confident.

Spend time in nature

Spending time in nature reduces stress, so take walks in nature whenever you can. Go forest bathing, and hug a tree. Whether you're deep in the wilderness or in a local park, feel your connection with nature through watching the birds, looking at fish in a pond or squirrels running up tree trunks. Nature can be a source of awe, whether you're looking at a huge sequoia or at tiny landscapes of lichen and moss on an old stump or stone.

Walk mindfully. I can go and walk round the block and come back and eat breakfast, and I've just had some physical exercise. Or I can go walk round the block mindfully, and notice the quality of the light today, a blackbird singing, contrails in the sky, the wind rising and then falling again, the fact that the apple blossom is coming out. I find that does me much more good. I'm also trying to keep my breathing nice and slow and stay aware of it, so my walking is a kind of walking meditation.

Sunshine is healthy; it gives your body the raw materials for vitamin D, and will help reduce the chance of you getting SAD (seasonal affective disorder). There's even a name for getting out in nature – 'ecotherapy' – and it has been shown to help with mild depression.

Volunteer

As well as connecting with nature, connect with other people. Volunteering is a good way to do this. You may find your purpose in helping others. You could volunteer for a food bank, charity shop, sports or arts organization, environmental cause, repair cafe, or faith-based cause, for instance. Volunteers often enjoy better physical and mental health, and have a feeling of meaningfulness and appreciation that comes to them through their work. In fact, older people who volunteer live longer than those who don't.

During the Covid lockdown, my local Sikh community organized food deliveries for immuno-suppressed people who couldn't get out shopping or didn't feel safe doing so. A colleague of mine joined in, who isn't a very 'conforming' Sikh, but he said it made a real difference to his life and actually helped him understand the community's values a lot better.

By nurturing relationships, volunteering makes it impossible to feel lonely. You might also learn new skills. And it doesn't have to take a huge amount of time. One of my friends volunteers every year for Crisis at Christmas, which looks after homeless people over the festive season. It's the one time of the year that he gets to cook – Christmas dinner for a couple of hundred people! I speak to an older gentleman who is lonely, through AgeUK every week. I have been doing this for five years now and would not stop it for anything. I get as much out of it as he does.

Foster animals

You might want to foster cats who need to get used to living with a family again before they find their forever home. You could use your professional skills, helping write press releases for a charity, or delivering IT or first-aid training to other volunteers. You could even volunteer with the whole family. A friend has volunteered with her family to house and look after a young Ukrainian refugee.

Eat chocolate

The last thing I'm going to mention here in this chapter is chocolate, and in particular, dark chocolate.

I may have a vested interest in believing it, but there is some evidence that cocoa polyphenols reduce stress. A piece of research in the *International Journal of Health Sciences* in 2014 was based on only a small group of subjects, but found out that "Consumption of 40 g of dark and milk chocolate daily during a period of two weeks appear to be an effective way to reduce perceived stress in females." White chocolate has no effect, showing that it's cocoa solids (which don't appear in white chocolate) which make the difference.

Watch out, though: chocolate is lovely, but commercial brands often contain a lot of added fat and sugar. Your healthiest best is cocoa powder, or intense, dark chocolate with a really high cocoa-solids content.

This chapter has taken you through a number of ways you can care for your body, mind, and soul. Take from it whatever sounds right for you. We are different, and everyone has their own particular ways of coping. The sole criterion for success is that you feel relaxed, grounded, and happy.

ACTION STEPS

1. Take some time to think about what areas of your life need a little TLC. Do you feel tired all the time, or stressed out? Do you somehow feel you're not achieving what you could? Do you feel lonely, or unattractive? Whatever negative feelings you have about yourself and your life, those are areas where you want to give yourself a little love.

2. Sit down with a piece of paper and plan your self-care regime; if that sounds too self-indulgent, call it 'regular maintenance.'

Some things, you might plan daily (meditation, coloring book, gratitude journal), others perhaps every weekend (nature walks, painting class), and some when you need them (long bath with aromatherapy oils, extra chocolate, hugs).

3. Get support from family/friends. Find things in your list that you can do together. If you have friends who practise meditation or yoga, for instance, ask them if they can help you get started.

4. Find a cause you could volunteer for. It needs to be something you care about. Be honest with yourself about how much time you can spare, and see if it will fit into your life.

5. Eat that chocolate sometimes. Be happy.

6. Make at least ten minutes every day of 'me time' for meditation or relaxation. You deserve it. And you *need* it, too.

I really do mean that last action point. This book may be specifically about gut health for women, but I think that our happiness and our gut health are in some ways very much the same thing. The healthier your digestive system, the happier you will be – and the happier you are, the better your digestion will be.

Getting there might be tough. You may find you've got to eat less of some foods you really like, and you may not particularly like doing the elimination diet, or really enjoy your first 5k run.

On the other hand, I hope you're going to have some great discoveries along the way. You could find new foods you'd never even thought of trying before, new sports, and better ways to relax. If you put the action points in this book into practice, you should conquer any issues with IBS or bloating, enjoy better health generally, and become a happier person too. That's a bit more than I promised at the start of the book, but you are welcome to the extra happiness!

Chapter 10
THE IMPORTANCE OF MOVING YOUR BODY AND GETTING GOOD SLEEP

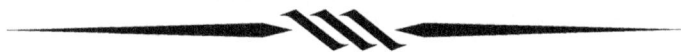

T his is the chapter you're not going to like.

I told you about diets and supplements and so on, and you thought "Great, I can do this." But it's not going to work unless you get up and do some exercise. And now you're quite likely thinking, "I don't have the time," or "I *hate* the gym," or "Running is kinda boring."

I am the kind of person who actually enjoys exercise, but I know that not everyone feels the same!

And I'm also going to tell you that you need to get some proper sleep... if you hated your parents telling you to go to bed way too early, then you're not going to enjoy that part of the chapter either.

But let's look at what exercise does for your body. It gets more oxygen going around, and that's good for your brain and your blood. You increase your core body temperature, too, and that's pretty good for your gut. Though scientists don't know exactly which mechanisms are at play, there's increasing research showing that adults who exercise regularly benefit from a more diverse and active gut microbiome.

Your body also needs good quality sleep, as well as the right number of hours.

Incorporating exercise into your life

Types of exercise

You need to get some good cardio-vascular exercise, three hours a week or so. This is the kind of exercise that gets you sweaty, makes your heart beat faster, and gets you out of breath. Most research looks at jogging or cycling, but it could include rowing, swimming, skipping, or dance.

You'll also want some exercise for stamina and strength, such as fixed or free weights, resistance training, squats, stretches, or Tai Chi. Your exercise program should be consistent, and you should try to exercise outdoors as much as you can. A Finnish study showed that children who play in the forest have better immune systems and gut microbiomes, as they're in touch with all kinds of microorganisms out there.

So okay, let's start working out how exactly you're going to get active, if you're not already!

There's no one way to do it. It's probably best to adopt a number of different types of exercise. I do free weights four times a week and my cardio is cycling once a week and circuits/interval training three times a week. I also do yoga a few times. One of my friends does a dance class, but she also runs, and swims every so often, usually when her kids want to go to the pool. Another friend hikes at the weekends, and during the week she does a couple of gym workouts before work. She loves the hiking, and regards the gym as "a necessary evil," she tells me. Since she discovered an outdoor gym installation in a local park, she's considering using that instead.

GREAT EXERCISES FOR GUT HEALTH

- Sit-ups, press-ups and crunches are great exercises for tightening up your abdomen, and this can help with gastric health. They increase the blood flow to your gastric tract, too. Plus, other than perhaps a good mat, you don't need any specialized equipment or clothing to do them. You'll want to do them on an empty stomach, though!

- Walking is great exercise, and again, doesn't need loads of gear to get started. Make sure you have comfortable shoes or trainers that give you adequate support, though. You'll want to walk briskly enough that you feel energized. If you enjoy being outside, you might want to try Nordic walking, where you use a pair of walking poles to get your whole body involved in swinging along.

- Yoga may benefit you if you're stressed out, as well as being good exercise. Many of the postures will help free up your abdomen and increase your centre strength, which can help your gut health by reducing some of the push and pull on your GI tract. Remember there are a number of different styles of yoga, so if you don't enjoy Bikram ('hot') yoga, which is performed in a strict sequence in a hot room, you might prefer Yin or restorative yoga, which is much softer in approach and focused on helping you feel refreshed and rejuvenated.

- Cycling is great exercise, although, obviously, you need a bicycle, and a good bike can be expensive. It's a cardio exercise which will get your heart rate up and improve your breathing, and if you live in an attractive area, it's a great way of getting outdoors. You may be lucky enough to live in a bike-friendly city – Amsterdam and Copenhagen are often mentioned, but the top cities in the US include Minneapolis; Portland, Oregon; Ann Arbor; Santa Monica; and Washington DC!

- Dance! There are plenty of fitness-orientated dance classes, from Zumba to aerobic dance, or you could take up a traditional dance style. The important thing is to enjoy it and to get moving, and take friends along – or make friends while you're there. If you love music and rhythm, add dance to your exercise roster. Twists and turns are great for your abs.

- Team sports aren't for everyone, but if you enjoy soccer, netball, baseball, or other sports, get stuck in. A good team will always have a stretch and workout before playing, which will really help your general health. If competitive frisbee is more your thing, that's fine too!

One kind of very specific exercise which can help with all kinds of digestive/ gastric issues is pelvic floor exercises, such as Kegel exercises. These are particularly useful for women who often have incontinence after childbirth – in France, new mothers are taught to do these exercises for several months after the birth to get back into condition – but they work for men, too. If you imagine the muscles you need to use when you're desperately trying *not* to pee, or *not* to fart – those are exactly the muscles you're going to exercise. Tighten those muscles for three seconds, then relax them for three seconds – that's one Kegel. Do a set (ten to fifteen kegels) every morning and every evening. You can extend the length of each cycle later, and do two sets instead of one; the important thing is that you should feel quite comfortable doing the exercise.

You might also decide to do workouts at home, and here, YouTube is your best friend, with a number of workouts aimed at abdominal health. Simply choose the approach and instructor closest to your style, play the video and follow along. I use YouTube for my yoga workouts.

Find what works for you. You have to enjoy it, for a start. My sister enjoys swimming, but if you're scared of the water, or just don't like the smell of chlorine, it's not going to be a good choice for you. First off, it's going to be that much extra effort to go and do your exercise, and when you've done it, you're not going to feel relaxed and happy. Try to choose something that won't bore you. That might mean getting outside for a hike, gamifying your exercise (Pokemon Go will get you out and about!), or a competitive sport like badminton or pickleball.

You should also vary the intensity of your exercise. Even if you're an athlete, you'll want to do some gentler exercise, perhaps alternating days of higher and lower intensity (one day trail running, yoga or swimming the next). You should also mix cardiovascular exercise – the kind that gets you sweaty and breathing hard – with sessions of weights or stretching for muscle strength and flexibility.

You may want to exercise solo. You might want to get an exercise buddy or two. Or you might want to join a more organized class, do Parkruns, or join a team. You might even consider a personal trainer to get you started. We're all different, so pick what works for you.

Things to consider

However, you should know that you can have too much of a good thing – and though we usually say that about tasty food and drink, it's true of exercise as well! Excessive exercise can actually give you real gut problems if your workouts are too long or too intense. Monash University research aimed to pinpoint just where things started going wrong, looking at twenty years of academic studies of this phenomenon, and found that two hours of 60% VO2 max was the threshold. 60% VO2 max is where you're consuming 60% of your maximum oxygen consumption. If you have a Fitbit or similar device, it will calculate that for you, but 60% is where you're beginning to feel your heart going quite a bit faster, breaking sweat, and breathing hard. That's a good place to be, but not for too long, and if you start feeling under pressure or hurting from the exercise, it's time to slacken off.

Overexertion can damage your GI tract. It causes your intestinal cells to leak endotoxins, and you could then end up with 'leaky gut.' So be gentle when you start exercising, and don't get addicted to long workouts.

If you do exercise hard, it's worth taking a probiotic supplement. If you do HIIT (high intensity interval training), your body will experience some inflammation as a result of the exercise. However, if you take a probiotic, it will handle the inflammation and in doing so it will actually boost your body's immune system. This is how I counteract my HIIT.

Mindful exercise should help. Some of us tend to go to the gym, put our headphones on, and zone out while we torment our bodies. That's not really a great attitude to exercise. Even if you can't get out in the forest to hike, smell the scent of pine, listen to birdsong, and fill your lungs with wonderful clean air, you can try to make your exercise a more mindful experience. Pay attention to your body and how it feels, get into a good rhythm, and have a proper wind-down process to feel the benefits and remind yourself how much good you're doing by taking that exercise.

In your entire life, and particularly in your exercise, it's a good rule to do things that make you happy. It's scientifically proven that there is a link between good intestinal health and happiness. Ninety percent of our serotonin, a mood-regulating chemical that makes us feel happy, is produced by cells in our intestines, and the gut microbiome helps to regulate our serotonin. Comparisons of the microbiomes of depressed patients with a control group shows that those who were depressed had significant imbalances of bacteria in their gut. The 'microbiome-gut-brain axis' should be in balance; the beneficial effects are then multi-directional. A good microbiome helps you be happy, but equally, being happy will help you keep your gut microbiota in good order!

Yoga

I already mentioned yoga as an exercise option, but I strongly advocate it as an excellent stress release and relaxation experience, too. If you are a worrier, someone who is stressed out, or who finds it hard to let go, yoga can really help, as it focuses on breathing and mindfulness as well as physical exercise.

In particular, twisting postures can help relax your center and improve your digestion, and there are a number of postures that should help your digestive organs:

YOGA POSES

- *Uttanasana*, standing forward bend. You bend as far forward as you can, trying to put your face against your legs, and bring your hands round to grasp your ankles from behind.

- *Ushtrasana* or camel pose is almost the opposite, and stretches your abdominal region. Kneeling, you reach back to grasp your ankles, push your chest forward and let your head fall back.

- *Savasana*, corpse pose. This is the ultimate anti-stress pose. Lie on your back, let your feet flop outwards, and rest your arms a little way out from your body, with your palms facing up. Close your eyes, and breathe deeply. This is a good pose to use at the end of a session, to get the maximum relaxation.

- *Reclined butterfly*, lying down with your legs bent and the soles together. You can feel your thigh muscles stretch!

- *Parsva sukhanasa*, side bend. Sit cross-legged, and touch the floor with your hands at your sides. Raise your left arm right up, and lean to your right, stretching your left side. Then do it the other way around. Take it nice and slow and feel your obliques and belly muscles stretching and relaxing.

- *Apanasana* or wind-relieving pose. Lie on your back, then bring up your knees and hug them to your belly – both knees together, then one at a time. This is good for relaxing your colon.

- *Balasana* or child's pose is wonderfully relaxing. Kneel, then press your bottom into your heels but stretch the rest of your body forward and push your arms right out along the mat.

- *Vipaseet karani* - lie close to the wall and 'walk' your legs up the wall till they are stretched out vertically, then relax! The wall will do all the work.

- A combination of two poses helps stretch your back and belly muscles – cat and cow (*Marjaryasana, Bitilasana*). The basis for both poses is to start on your hands and knees, keeping your spine straight and flat. To get into cow pose, push your tailbone up and your belly will go down; roll your shoulders back and look upward, so you're in a U-shape. Hold that for a few breaths, go back into neutral, then become a cat by tucking in your tailbone and arching your back, like a cat that's about to hiss. Let your head fall gently downwards, too . So you're going from U to N, from convex to concave.

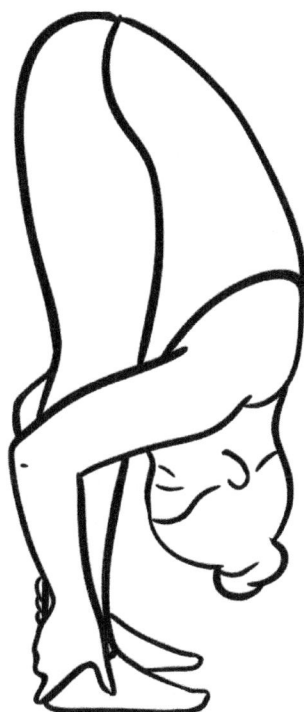

Uttanasana

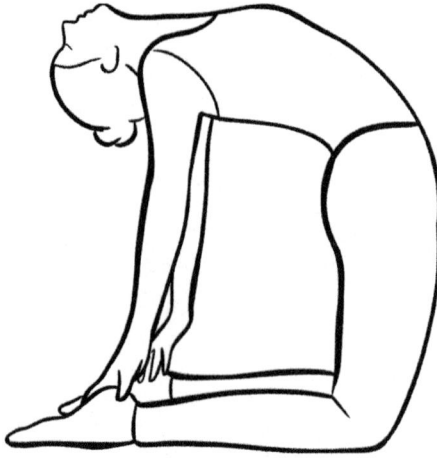

Ushtrasana

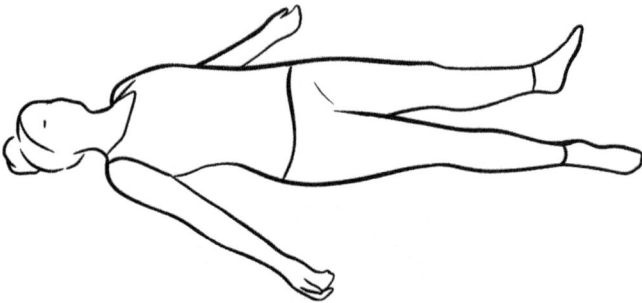

Savasana

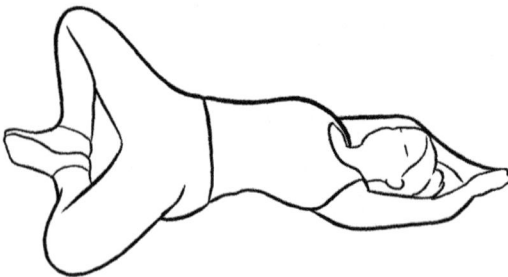

Reclined butterfly

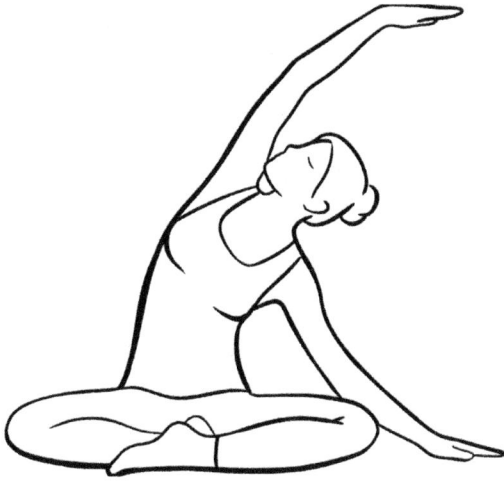

Parsva sukhanasa

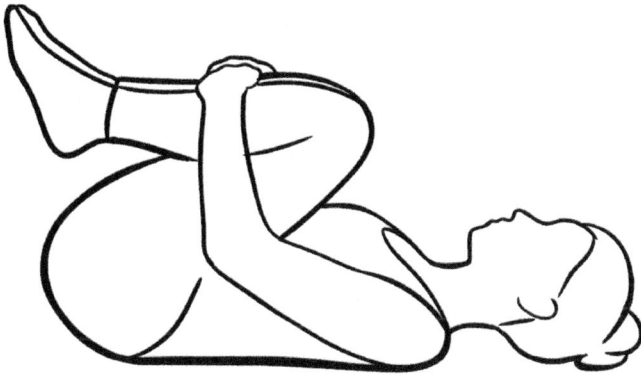

Apanasana

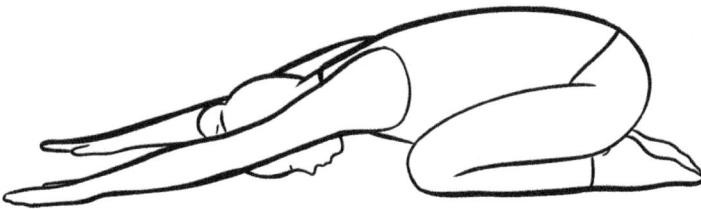

Balasana

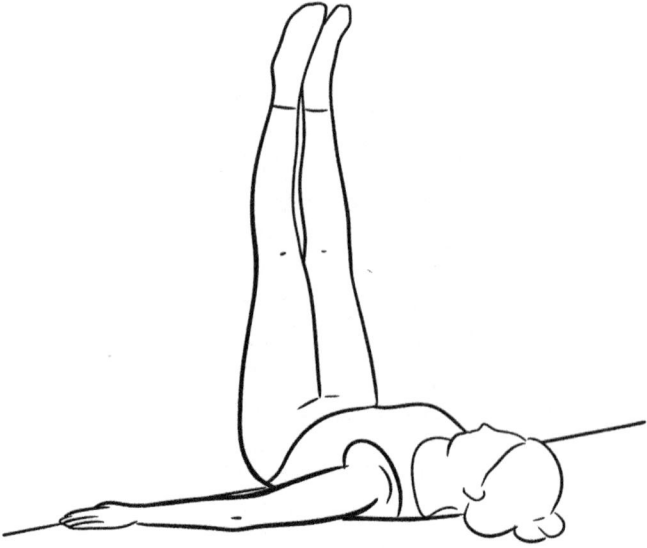

Vipaseet karani

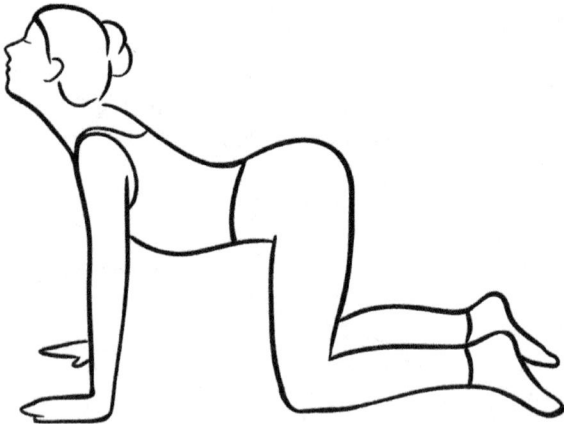

Marjaryasana

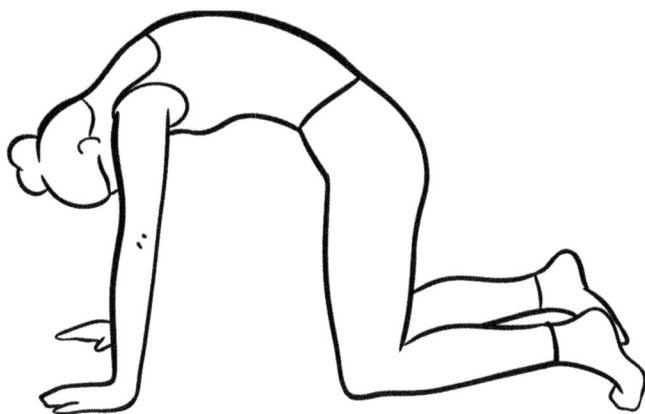

Bitilasana

However, don't get competitive at yoga. I've experienced some yoga studios where there's a really competitive vibe between some of the practitioners, particularly related to advanced *asanas* (postures), and that's both stressful and likely to result in strain or even injury.

Taking a break or taking it easy

Remember that even though physical exercise should become a continuous habit, it's fine to take a break from time to time. You might need to do so in order to heal, if you've been injured, or have a flare-up, or if you just feel tired and feel that you've overdone things. Or you might just need to call a halt half way through your usual 5k or half hour of circuit training, and say enough's enough.

You might want to take a break from exercise when work gets heavy (like accountants coming up to tax day), to prepare for an examination, or to take a vacation. Or you might just feel a bit fed up with what you're doing for exercise and want a break for a while to make other things a priority for a while. You don't need to worry about becoming unfit; it takes two months of inactivity to lose all your fitness gains. In fact, you'll only see a steep decline in your fitness if you're a really top athlete or extremely fit; most of us just lose a little bit of sharpness.

It's also okay to take tiny steps. You may find it useful to have the image of a woman warrior in your mind – a tall, fit, fast spear-carrier who can surge out of the pack – but it's actually *okay* to be jogging along at the back of the pack. If you have led a pretty sedentary life and you actually start walking half a mile a day, that's progress, and it's really going to do you good; if the woman next door runs marathons, so what? Don't judge yourself by others, just do the best you can for your own body and your own health.

By the way, endurance athletes really do need a break from time to time. There's a certain endurance mindset that can get you putting in longer and longer hours, and at a certain point, this can result in fatigue and 'overtraining.' That's why marathon runners usually *decrease* their training hours in the couple of weeks just before the race.

Do you *need* a break or are you just feeling a bit lazy? The way to tell is to listen to your body and be mindful of your own feelings.

- Do you really dread your workouts, rather than just not feeling particularly enthusiastic?
- Do you have a sore or painful joint, aches and pains that won't go away?
- Are you feeling physically exhausted and drained?

If any of these apply to you, you actually do need a break. On the other hand, if you're just bored with, say, training for a running event, maybe you just need to mix up your exercise regime a bit more and do some dance, practise yoga, go snorkeling, or have a kickabout – something to get away from worrying about your pace and halfway splits.

When you come back from a break, of course, remember to take things gently. Give your body time to readjust, start with the simplest exercises, take a rest a few times during your routine, and take some extra rest days if you need them.

Reducing stress through exercise

As we discussed in the previous chapter, you should try and minimize too much stress in your life. Stressful events tend to evoke a 'fight or flight' response, and that means your adrenal gland will create cortisol and push it out into your bloodstream. A small amount of cortisol is fine; too much of it, and your body is struggling. You end up pumping out cortisol all the time, which results in high blood sugar, feeling hungry all the time (which can cause you to put on weight), digestive problems, a compromised immune system, and even heart problems (because cortisol narrows your arteries and increases your heart rate). It can also impact the hormones needed for a healthy reproductive system.

Fortunately, exercise can help reduce adrenaline and cortisol (possibly not if your preferred outdoors activities are paintball and bungee jumping, though!). Instead, it will help your body produce endorphins, which are natural painkillers and can heighten your mood. Endorphins are responsible for the 'runner's high.'

As well as taking physical exercise, try to relax properly. A good way to relax is to lie down or sit comfortably, and then focus on each group of muscles in turn – your forehead and eyes, your face, your jaws, your neck, chest, stomach, thighs, then your arms and hands, then your legs and feet. Tense up, then let go. Feel any aches and pains, and let them go. This should take ten minutes to a quarter of an hour, and should leave you feeling relaxed and unstressed. Do it twice a day for best results.

Exercise as a lifestyle

By the way, if you are motivated by improving your figure as well as having a healthier gut, remember that exercise on its own is not going to ensure you lose weight. In fact, what you eat, and how much you eat, has more to do with your weight than how much you exercise. You need to be burning more calories than you eat, so if you exercise more but also eat more, you won't necessarily get rid of the pounds, though you *will* be fitter.

The 80/20 rule applies here: diet usually gives you 80% of your weight loss and exercise is just responsible for 20%. It's much easier to cut out 400 calories from your diet – that's one and a half Pop Tarts or a brownie – than it is to lose that weight through exercise. You'd have to swim for forty-five minutes, or run quite fast for half an hour, to do that, and on a bike it might take you an hour or more.

But of course, eating right and not taking exercise could make you skinny, unfit, and unhappy. So it's important to get both things in the right proportion!

While your lifestyle may mean you don't have a lot of choice about when to exercise, if you can choose, think about when is your best time. For me, it's always the morning, as that's a great mood booster, particularly in summer, when I can get out early and greet the sunrise. Find the part of the day when you have the most energy, and feel active and enthusiastic. You may find you have two bursts of energy, one in the morning and one in the early evening, let's say. Or you may find that you're tetchy and unenthusiastic in the morning, but in the mid-afternoon, you have that sweet spot when you feel great and have plenty of energy. Try to make use of that time to exercise; it will be easier to motivate yourself and you'll get better results and enjoy yourself more. Since the Covid pandemic, employers are much more flexible with the hours you work or when you take your breaks; take advantage of these changes in flexibility.

But what if formal exercise really turns you off? Or what if you don't have a block of time you can devote to jogging or the gym or a yoga class? There are all kinds of ways you can build a bit more exercise into your daily routine. Park a bit further from work, or in the far corner of the supermarket parking lot, so you have to walk a bit more. Take the stairs instead of the lift (though not if you work on the 31st floor, obviously). Go for a walk outside at lunchtime or before you take the car home, if you work on a campus with some nice paths.

Even just getting up from your desk every so often and walking down the corridor can help you keep active. Go to see people you're engaged in projects with, rather than phoning or emailing them. Don't get lunch delivered and eat it at your desk; go out to get your lunch, or head for the canteen.

When you get up, just do some quick stretches in your bedroom or bathroom. If you have a dog, let it help you exercise a bit, or help walk a neighbor's dog from time to time! Keep some free weights in the house and do a bit of lifting while you watch TV.

You can even do chair yoga! Okay, maybe this is really best if you work at home, but quite a lot of the postures won't get noticed in the office. You can try a seated version of the cow-cat stretch I mentioned earlier, just making sure you curve your spine both different ways; that will help make sure you don't get back-ache! You can twist to the right and left while you're sitting on your chair, too. Taking chair yoga further can be a great way to exercise if you have mobility issues or are recovering from illness.

To finish the day, I like to do yoga at bedtime. It's not just exercise; it helps me get nicely relaxed so that I can enjoy a full night's sleep. I manage to fall asleep practically as soon as my head hits the pillow! Poses such as the reclined butterfly, where you lie down with your legs bent and the soles together, or the 'corpse pose' (I do wish it was called something nicer!) are really good. Take it slowly, breathe deeply, and feel the energy in your body.

Child's pose (*balasana*) is also a great bedtime asana. You might also enjoy *vipaseet karani* – both listed in yoga poses earlier in the chapter.

If you've followed this chapter faithfully, you know how important exercise is to your health, but you should also have a good feeling for the kind of exercise you will enjoy.

Sleeping well

You may have found that one of the problems of an unhealthy lifestyle was not getting enough sleep, or perhaps, getting eight hours' sleep but not actually feeling rested when you woke up in the morning. Lack of sleep is often associated with poor gut health, so you should already be getting better sleep once you've taken up your new diet, but this is something that cuts two ways: if you're not sleeping well, your gut microbiome might suffer. So let's see how you can get a better night's sleep.

Better sleep can help you avoid a blood sugar spike right after breakfast and a subsequent dip a couple of hours later. That means you won't get mid-morning munchies, something which has a lot of people reaching for the cookie jar.

Better sleep should also help reduce your stress levels. Higher stress increases the amount of cortisol, a stress hormone, in your body, and this in turn can impact on the gut microbiome. Better sleep will also create more melatonin, which helps you fall asleep, and also helps regulate your GI system. In particular, melatonin stops acid reflux.

Stress can also impact your sleep patterns, and sleep rhythms are connected to how your gut works. You should ideally be sleeping seven to nine hours, but the American average is below seven hours, so a lot of people are not getting enough sleep. Over 40% of Americans report having sleep issues, or stress keeping them awake at night. At its worst, a vicious circle develops: stress means you don't get enough sleep, and then not having enough sleep makes you stressed.

Studies by the American Psychological Association show that people sleeping fewer than eight hours a night are most likely to report symptoms of stress. Many say they're not getting enough sleep because their minds race. Others say they feel sluggish during the day.

Finally, if you're feeling tired all the time, that often means you'll end up with cravings for the wrong kinds of food – really sugary food, trans fats, processed foods. Think how often you've had unhealthy fast food because you felt too tired to cook or just want a sugar rush to stay awake.

So improving your sleep is something you ought to be doing. One thing that should help with both sleeping and GI health is not eating too late. If you eat just before you go to bed, you'll be trying to sleep and digest at the same time, and your body isn't designed for that.

Ways to improve your sleep

You can really help improve your sleep by having a nightly routine. Follow the same steps each night; this gets your brain to fall into the habit of getting ready for sleep. Take twenty minutes or so to wind down; listen to some music, do some relaxation exercises, or a little stretching (but not aerobic exercise), or read something that's not connected with your work and that helps you relax, like a good novel.

Get your body ready for sleep. For instance, do some slow stretches before you go to bed. This will make you more aware of your body, and develop mindfulness, but it also helps you relax. Give yourself a bear hug! Or do gentle neck stretches, looking behind you each side, dropping your head down then raising it again, or doing 'head rolls' – go very gently and stop if it becomes painful. You could do the child's pose from the yoga exercises.

Watch out for the impact of caffeine! Some people live in a whirl of not getting enough sleep, then relying on energy drinks and coffee to keep them going all day. Stop caffeine eight hours before bedtime, or even earlier. Keeping a caffeine diary the way you kept a food diary can be helpful.

Before bed, take a drink that can help you relax and sleep well. Cherry juice includes tryptophan, an amino acid that can help make melatonin, the chemical that helps regulate your sleep; drink two cups a day (this doesn't necessarily have to be at bedtime). Chamomile tea is a folk remedy, and not scientifically proven, but lots of people find this infusion beneficial (by the way, it doesn't actually contain tea). Ashwagandha and valerian teas are also often recommended, but both of these are more likely to cause problems such as headache, dizziness and dry mouth (note that valerian must not be taken with alcohol).

Peppermint tea is another good infusion. It is able to ease stomach pain, if that is stopping you sleeping. Make sure, if you use these infusions, to leave the bag soaking for ten minutes or so in the boiling water; don't just dip the tea bag in and out.

A cup of warm milk makes a soothing ritual just before bed. You could try 'golden milk' with turmeric, ginger and honey infused in the milk.

Build in a daily electronics detox. No Twitter, Facebook, instant messaging, or playing video games for the last half hour of the day. Dim the lights a little while before you aim to sleep. Try to have a regular time to turn in – it really helps. Ten minutes either side doesn't matter particularly, but if you're going to bed some nights at ten, and others at midnight, your body won't know what to expect.

Doomscrolling, catching up with email, or playing Candy Crush, will all put your sleep in peril. First of all, these are not great ways to relax, as they'll keep your mind active. Watching TV in bed is also not a great idea; if you want a really healthy life, move your TV to the living room. Secondly, electronic devices emit blue light, which can reduce the natural production of melatonin. It can also reduce the proportion of your sleep time spent in slow-wave and REM (rapid eye movement) sleep, which are the two most important stages of sleep as far as your brain is concerned.

So using an electronic device can mean you take longer to get to sleep, and when you do get to sleep, you'll get a lower quality of sleep as well.

You might want to read a little before you sleep. If you have an e-reader or tablet, it may have a blue light reduction or nighttime mode setting, so use that to keep the 'bad' light to a minimum. You should also keep your bedroom lighting low as you prepare for sleep; this sends a message to your brain that it's time to produce melatonin and get ready for sleeping. It might be better to listen to an audiobook rather than read.

The right color of light is important for good sleep. Red, orange, and yellow are conducive to sleep, which is one reason most night lights are red. You can also use laser lights to diffuse colored lights through the room, even playing a starscape of the whole galaxy on the walls of your room.

Meditating before sleep is a good idea. A 2015 study analyzed meditation's effect on patients with insomnia, and found that those who meditated reported better sleep. Meditation can increase the release of melatonin, increase serotonin, reduce the heart rate, and reduce blood pressure.

Don't 'try to go to sleep.' By making sleep a success and not sleeping a failure, that introduces stress just when you need to relax! Try to relax instead. Breathe deeply, feel if there is any stress or muscle tension in your body, and relax it. Having a relaxation MP3 play gently in the background, or using a particular song that you associate with bedtime, may help.

If, after twenty minutes, you feel relaxed but you're not asleep, get up and read a book for a while. Don't lie in bed feeling frustrated. Your body should associate being in bed with sleeping; that's why you should get up if you're not asleep. After you've read for a little while, you may be ready for sleep.

Sometimes you just need to get your sleeping quarters better organized. Your pillow may not be comfortable; if you sleep on your side, for instance, you may need a harder pillow for support. If your mattress creaks or has lumps, it's time to get a new one. Some people sleep 'hot,' warming up fast; if you're like this, but you don't like sleeping with very thin sheets, a weighted blanket can help you feel 'hugged' and protected while being thin enough that you don't overheat. Other people need the bed warmed up before they get in, or they shiver for ages. That's me!

Another thing that makes getting good sleep much easier is to try to get a regular bedtime every night. Regularity will help your body and nervous system get ready automatically. Make your wake-up time regular, too. Often, we try to adjust for being late to bed one night by having a lie-in the next morning, but that can lead to getting into a vicious spiral of going to bed later and later. In fact, if you're a night-owl, you may find it easier to set your wake-up time first, so that you get tired enough during the day that your body wants to go to sleep at the right time.

If you get good sleep, your entire body is going to benefit. And if you also practise intermittent fasting by taking a latish breakfast and an early dinner, you will be resting your gut properly, and giving it the break it needs from continual digestion so it can clean itself and prepare for the day ahead.

Other things that can help include:

- Heavier curtains, or an eye mask to block out light from outside.

- Ear plugs or a white noise machine to ensure you're not bothered by outside noise.

- A daylight lamp alarm which will mimic a natural sunrise to wake you gently, particularly when the mornings are still dark when it's time to go to work.

- Calming aromatherapy scents such as lavender, jasmine, and vanilla, in a diffuser, or added to your bath if you have a soak before bedtime.

Good sleep is a habit, and one that it's possible to acquire. If you have tried out all these suggestions and you still have problems sleeping, it may be worth talking to your doctor.

WAYS TO GET BETTER SLEEP

- Get into a habit of winding down before you go to bed – listen to music, do some relaxation exercises, do some stretches, read a book, do some gentle yoga.
- Don't drink caffeine before bed.
- Have a drink that will help you relax – cherry juice, chamomile tea, ashwagandha and valerian teas, peppermint tea, warm milk, golden milk.
- Build in an electronics detox.
- Have the right color lights – red, orange and yellow.
- Meditate.
- Don't force sleep; try to relax.
- See if your sleeping quarters need reorganizing.
- Have a regular bedtime.

How meditation can help

We tend to think that some people are calm while others are worriers, get flustered, or don't have much confidence. But in fact, calm and serenity – like good sleep – are habits that are not difficult to acquire.

If you haven't been taught how to meditate, the easiest way to start is just to focus on your breathing. You can use an app to set the time – start with just three minutes, then over time you can increase the length of your meditation up to ten or twenty minutes. Breathe slowly. For instance, you might take ten counts to breathe in, ten to hold your breath, ten to exhale. You might also use an app like Headspace, Calm or Buddhify.

Guided imagery for calmness is one way of dealing with stress, but it brings its benefits even if you don't feel particularly stressed out. Just ten minutes of guided imagery can really help you, and can lower your cholesterol and glucose levels as well as stress and anxiety. Start by breathing slowly and regularly, thinking of a peaceful place – a seaside walk, a beautiful cathedral, a mountain top or the middle of a forest. It can be a real place you have experienced, or an imagined place.

Think of details in the scene, the sounds and sensations – tastes, smells, how you are feeling. If you see or hear anything you don't like – a snake in the forest, for instance – just change where you are: go back a little way and branch off the track, or go somewhere else. Find a path to walk along, and relax.

When you have found your happy place, remember it for later. The more often you visit, and the better you know it and can imagine it, the more useful it is, because it will become a safe space that you can quickly access any time that you feel you need support or relaxation. You might want to associate it with a possession like a stone or a bracelet that you can carry with you; that gives you the ability to summon it (just like magic!) by touching your amulet.

At the end of your visit return, gently, to this world, feel where you are, make sure you feel grounded, and then open your eyes. You won't need to take more than ten or fifteen minutes. If you find it difficult visualizing your own spaces, use an app like Creative Space, Headspace, Guided Imagery, or Simply Being.

Another kind of self-care uses the power of touch – hugs. I know people who sign off emails 'hugs xxxx,' but even so, I think we grossly underestimate the power of a hug. It can be incredibly powerful as encouragement or congratulation or support. Make sure to celebrate 21 January – National Hugging Day!

Hugging can reduce stress, relieve pain, and reduce anxiety. If you have a huggy lifestyle, you'll have an improved immune system and healthier heart. Kids who grow up being hugged are happier than those who childhood is spent in a more distanced family. Added to which, hugging releases oxytocin, a chemical that enhances trust and bonding.

If no one else is around, you can even give yourself a hug!

ACTION STEPS

1. Make a list of activities and sports that appeal to you or that you'd like to try out. You might remember games that were fun when you were a child, or you might have seen something on TV last week. Promise yourself you'll give them a try!

2. Try listening to your body for a whole day. What's it telling you? Is your breathing really shallow? Are your shoulders or back aching? Do you feel a lack of energy? Do you feel stressed?

3. Start gently with a mindful walk in the park. Be aware of your body but also be aware of what's around you – the air, birdsong, other people, plants, sun or clouds, and so on. Let yourself be inspired.

4. Try out two or three different new activities, or more if you can. Many exercise classes let you sign up for a taster lesson without having to subscribe, so you're not taking a big risk.

5. Get a feel for what mix of activities and environments is good for

you. Draft yourself a daily or weekly schedule. And get going!

6. Keep a sleep diary for a couple of weeks. Note when you went to bed, when you woke up, how you slept. Note if you woke up during the night and how long (roughly) it took you to get to sleep again. Are you sleeping well, just about okay, or badly? If you're not sleeping well, it's time to take action.

Conclusion

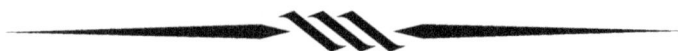

I started this book looking inside the human body, at your gut, and then at the trillions of microorganisms that live there and help to keep you healthy. It's a whole miniature universe, of which you are the master (if you want to be) or possibly the victim (if you don't). And it's more important to the whole body than you might think. The gut is connected with the brain, and it's also one of the big factors that keep your immune system strong, so if your gut isn't healthy, you're likely to feel it elsewhere too.

I also talked about why women really need to know about gut health. IBS is a huge problem for women, not just because our bodies are arranged in a different way from men's, but because we have so much work and stress thrown at us that looking after our health is often the last thing on our agendas. Plus we are meant to be more in tune with our gut!

The remaining chapters were based on things I found out during my own struggle against IBS. First, I learned how using an elimination diet established which foods made me feel ill or bloated, so that I could cut them out of my life. To be honest, the diet was difficult, but it made such a big difference when I finally found out what was triggering my IBS, the result was well worth the ordeal.

The next chapter covered how to detox in order to give your body a week or two of rest and recuperation from what you've been putting it through. This is always a good idea from time to time, just like changing the oil in a car or giving the house a spring clean. And then there's the ongoing work of making sure my diet contains the right prebiotics and probiotics to keep my gut microbiome in balance, and taking exercise that not only keeps me healthy, but keeps my abdomen in good order.

Finally, I talked about the self-care that can fully actualize your happiness – something I'm still working on!

As you followed along, I hope you made a start on the action points at the end of each chapter. If you have, you should already have seen some beneficial changes to your life, and you are well on your way to having a happy and healthy gut.

I like to keep my books up to date and I'm always interested in what readers have to say, so I'd be really grateful if you'd give the book a review on Amazon. It helps me make the next edition even more useful if I know what did work, and what didn't, or if I need to be more specific in certain areas. It helps other readers to find the book too.

Gut Health Secrets for Women: Share the Glow of Wellness

Now that you've uncovered the keys to achieving optimum gut health, it's time to pay it forward and guide others to the same radiant well-being.

By sharing your honest thoughts about Gut Health Secrets for Women on Amazon, you're not just leaving a review; you're illuminating the path for fellow women seeking the wisdom and empowerment found within these pages. Your words can spark their passion for gut health and guide them to the wellness they've been searching for.

Thank you for being a vital part of this chain of knowledge. The glow of gut health stays ablaze when we pass on our insights, and you're playing a crucial role in preserving and nurturing it.

Scan the QR code below to leave your review (just so you know, this takes you to the review page of Amazon US, if you live in a different country, simply change the .com to the relevant country domain suffix. Or you can go to your order page to leave a review there):

Your contribution means the world. Together, we're fostering a community of empowered individuals, and your review is a beacon guiding others toward the same enlightenment.

With heartfelt gratitude, Naomi Olson

PS - Remember, your review isn't just a comment; it's a gift of guidance for someone else. Scan the QR code above to share the glow of wellness.

Glossary

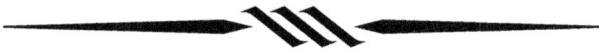

Antibiotics – drugs that can block the growth of bacteria (but not viruses): also called antibacterials

Antigen – a substance that activates the production of antibodies.

Antibody – produced by your immune system when it detects something in your body that should not be there, like a virus or antigen. Antibodies recognize specific antigens and will latch on to them.

Autoimmune disorder – any disease which involves 'false alarms' from your immune system, when it confuses your healthy body tissues for antigens, and attacks them.

Bacteria – microorganisms that live in a relationship with a plant or animal (including humans). They may be symbiotic, that is, mutually beneficial, or parasitic, or simply 'commensal' (using the same food supply). Some can be harmful, but many are not; in fact, many of them are essential for our health.

Bile – a liquid created by your liver that helps you digest fats.

Bloating – swelling of the abdomen provoked by excess gas. It can cause pain in the belly, often mild but sometimes intensely painful.

Bifidobacteria or bifidus – a kind of bacteria that naturally lives in a mammal's gut, and that you can also find in fermented foods such as yogurt.

Clostridium difficile – a species of bacteria that is not problematic in a healthy gut, but can cause problems if there is an imbalance. Such an imbalance is often caused by antibiotic treatments.

Commensal – organisms that 'share a table,' in other words, share a food source without having any other relationship with each other.

Crohn's disease – a type of inflammatory bowel disease that can affect any part of the digestive system. Symptoms include abdominal pain, diarrhea, and fatigue. It may become worse over time, and may also exhibit a pattern of intermittent flare-ups separated by periods of remission.

Cytokine – a protein that has an effect on the immune system.

Dysbiosis/dysbacteriosis – an imbalance of microbial colonies in the human body, e.g., in mucous membranes, or in the gut.

Enterotype – a stable cluster of bacterial communities, of which three types appear to exist, linked to different types of diet. However, researchers are still evaluating the data and assessing how exactly these enterotypes work.

Eschericia coli (E. coli) – this bacteria species hits the news regularly as a dangerous cause of disease. However, most E. coli strains are harmless and live naturally in the gut.

Fecal microbiota transplantation – this procedure has been used effectively on patients suffering from C.difficile infection,, but its general use has not been authorized.

Fermentation – the conversion of sugars and carbohydrates into an acid or alcohol by a microorganism such as yeast; used to make pickles, beer, wine, yogurt, or bread, for instance.

Gastrointestinal (GI) tract – all your organs involved in the consumption, digestion and excretion of food, from the mouth to the anus.

Gut flora – an old-fashioned way of referring to the bacterial community living in the gut; microbiota (Greek for 'small life') is more accurate.

Gut microbiota – the community of microorganisms living in the gut, made up of many different kinds of microbes.

Immune system – the body's defence system against infectious organisms; the immune response, acting through a cascade of biological reactions, acts to eliminate the detected agent.

Inflammatory bowel disease – occurs when the wall of one section of the digestive tract becomes swollen; can include Crohn's disease and ulcerative colitis.

Inflammation – a natural response by the body when it needs to fight against an aggression. May be characterized by redness, heat, pain, or by an organ's normal functioning being affected.

Irritable bowel syndrome (IBS) – a common disorder affecting 15-20% of people; more common in women than in men.

Lactobacillus – this bacteria normally inhabits the gut, and is found in fermented foods like yogurt. Lactobacilli can help in treating diarrhea.

Metabolite – a small molecule made when the body breaks down food.

Metagenome – the entire collection of microbial genes found in a particular environment.

Microbial ecology – the study of the interaction between microbes and the environment.

Microbiota – microorganisms that reside on or inside the human body.

Microbiome – the entire collection of genes found in the microbiota.

Microorganism – microscopic organisms including fungi, viruses, and bacteria.

NSAID – Non-steroidal anti-inflammatory drugs, such as drugs taken for arthritis and similar chronic conditions. Common painkiller Nurofen/ Ibuprofen is an NSAID.

Pathogen – an infectious biological agent (e.g., a virus or bacteria) that can produce a disease in its host.

PCOS - Polycystic ovary syndrome, or pelvic congestion syndrome, which can cause chronic pelvic pain.

Prebiotic – food components such as fiber that are non-digestible but stimulate the activity of particular bacterial groups (e.g., lactobacilli, bifidobacteria), and can have a beneficial effect on gut health.

Probiotic – live microorganisms which can help balance the gut micobiome, consumed in supplements or with fermented foods such as kimchi, yogurt or kefir.

Symbiosis – a relationship between two organisms which need each other in order to survive. Gut bacteria couldn't live without us, and we can't live without them.

Bibliography

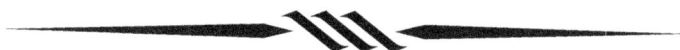

Amato, K. R., Arrieta, M. C., Azad, M. B., et al. (2021). The human gut microbiome and health inequities. Proceedings of the National Academy of Sciences of the United States of America, 118(25), e2017947118. https://doi.org/10.1073/pnas.2017947118

Benedict, C., Vogel, H., Jonas, W., Woting, A., Blaut, M., Schürmann, A., & Cedernaes, J. (2016). Gut microbiota and glucometabolic alterations in response to recurrent partial sleep deprivation in normal-weight young individuals. Molecular Metabolism, 5(12), 1175-1186. https://doi.org/10.1016/j.molmet.2016.10.003

Clarke, S. F., Murphy, E. F., O'Sullivan, O., Lucey, A. J., Humphreys, M., Hogan, A., Hayes, P., O'Reilly, M., Jeffery, I. B., Wood-Martin, R., Kerins, D. M., Quigley, E., Ross, R. P., O'Toole, P. W., Molloy, M. G., Falvey, E., Shanahan, F., Cotter, P. D. (2014). Exercise and associated dietary extremes impact on gut microbial diversity. Gut, 63(12), 1913-1920. https://doi.org/10.1136/gutjnl-2013-306541

Dewulf, E. M., Cani, P. D., Claus, S. P., Fuentes, S., Puylaert, P. G., Neyrinck, A. M., Bindels, L. B., de Vos, W. M., Gibson, G. R., Thissen, J. P., Delzenne, N. M. (2013). Insight into the prebiotic concept: lessons from an exploratory, double blind intervention study with inulin-type fructans in obese women. Gut, 62(8), 1112-1121. https://doi.org/10.1136/gutjnl-2012-303304

Donohoe, D. R., Garge, N., Zhang, X., O'Connell, T. M., Bunger, M., Bultman, S. J. (2011). The Microbiome and Butyrate Regulate Energy Metabolism and Autophagy in the Mammalian Colon. Cell Metabolism, 13(5), 517–526. https://doi.org/10.1016/j.cmet.2011.02.018

EIGE. (2019). Gender Equality Index. EIGE. ISBN: 978-92-9482-382-3. DOI: 10.2839/319154

Grabrucker, S., et al. (2022). Faecal microbiota transplantation from Alzheimer's participants induces impairments in neurogenesis and cognitive behaviours in rats. bioRxiv, 2022.11.04.515189. https://doi.org/10.1101/2022.11.04.515189

Guo, Y., Qi, Y., Yang, X., Zhao, L., Wen, S., Liu, Y., et al. (2016). Association between Polycystic Ovary Syndrome and Gut Microbiota. PLoS ONE, 11(4), e0153196. https://doi.org/10.1371/journal.pone.0153196

Gupta, S., Allen-Vercoe, E., Petrof, E. O. (2016). Fecal microbiota transplantation: in perspective. Therapeutic Advances in Gastroenterology, 9(2), 229-239. https://doi.org/10.1177/1756283X15607414

Gamage, H. K. A. H., Sathili, A. M. M., Nishtala, K., Chong, R. W. W., Packer, N. H., Paulsen, I. T. (2022). doi: https://doi.org/10.1101/2022.09.15.508181

Heiman, M. L., Greenway, F. L. (2016). A healthy gastrointestinal microbiome is dependent on dietary diversity. Molecular Metabolism, 5(5), 317-320. https://doi.org/10.1016/j.molmet.2016.02.005

Huerta-Franco, M. R., Vargas-Luna, M., Tienda, P., Delgadillo-Holtfort, I., Balleza-Ordaz, M., & Flores-Hernandez, C. (2013). Effects of occupational stress on the gastrointestinal tract. World Journal of Gastrointestinal Pathophysiology, 4(4), 108-118. https://doi.org/10.4291/wjgp.v4.i4.108

Kanen, J., Nazir, R., Sedky, K., Pradhan, B. K. (2015). The Effects of Mindfulness-Based Interventions on Sleep Disturbance: A Meta-Analysis. Adolescent Psychiatry, 5(2), 105-115.

Kelly, J. R., Borre, Y., O'Brien, C., Patterson, E., et al. (2016). Transferring the blues: Depression-associated gut microbiota induces neurobehavioural changes in the rat. Journal of Psychiatric Research, 82(5), 5-12. https://doi.org/10.1016/j.jpsychires.2016.07.019

Kim, Y. S., Kim, N. (2018). Sex-Gender Differences in Irritable Bowel Syndrome. Journal of Neurogastroenterology and Motility, 24(4), 544-558. https://doi.org/10.5056/jnm18082

Leeuwendaal, N. K., Stanton, C., O'Toole, P. W., Beresford, T. P. (2022). Fermented Foods, Health and the Gut Microbiome. Nutrients, 14(7), 1527. https://doi.org/10.3390/nu14071527

Miclotte, L., Van de Wiele, T. (2020). Food processing, gut microbiota and the globesity problem. Critical Reviews in Food Science and Nutrition, 60(11), 1769-1782. https://doi.org/10.1080/10408398.2019.1596878

Mitchell, S. J., Bernier, M., Mattison, J. A., et al. (2018). Daily Fasting Improves Health and Survival in Male Mice Independent of Diet Composition and Calories. Cell Metabolism. Advance online publication. https://doi.org/10.1016/j.cmet.2018.08.011

Monda, V., et al. (2017). Exercise Modifies the Gut Microbiota with Positive Health Effects. Oxidative Medicine and Cellular Longevity, 2017, 3831972. https://doi.org/10.1155/2017/3831972

Pan, X., Wen, S. W., Kaminga, A. C., et al. (2020). Gut metabolites and inflammation factors in non-alcoholic fatty liver disease: A systematic review and meta-analysis. Scientific Reports, 10, 8848. https://doi.org/10.1038/s41598-020-65051-8

Qin, Y., Havulinna, A. S., Liu, Y., Jousilahti, P., Ritchie, S. C., Tokolyi, A., Sanders, J. G., Valsta, L., Bro·y·ska, M., Zhu, Q., Tripathi, A., Vázquez-Baeza, Y., Loomba, R., Cheng, S., Jain, M., Niiranen, T., Lahti, L., Knight, R., Salomaa, V., Inouye, M., & Méric, G. (2022). Combined effects of host genetics and diet on human gut microbiota and incident disease in a single population cohort. Nature Genetics, 54(2), 134-142. https://doi.org/10.1038/s41588-021-00991-z

Roslund, M. I., et al. (2020). Biodiversity intervention enhances immune regulation and health-associated commensal microbiota among daycare children. Science Advances, 6, eaba2578. https://doi.org/10.1126/sciadv.aba2578

Rousseaux, C., Thuru, X., Gelot, A., Barnich, N., Neut, C., Dubuquoy, L., Dubuquoy, C., Merour, E., Geboes, K., Chamaillard, M., Ouwehand, A., Leyer, G., Carcano, D., Colombel, J. F., Ardid, D., & Desreumaux, P. (2007). Lactobacillus acidophilus modulates intestinal pain and induces opioid and cannabinoid receptors. Nature Medicine, 13(1), 35-37. https://doi. org/10.1038/nm1521

Rusch, H. L., Rosario, M., Levison, L. M., Olivera, A., Livingston, W. S., Wu, T., & Gill, J. M. (2019). The effect of mindfulness meditation on sleep quality: A systematic review and meta-analysis of randomized controlled trials. Annals of the New York Academy of Sciences, 1445(1), 5-16. https://doi. org/10.1111/nyas.13996

Shil, A., & Chichger, H. (2021). Artificial Sweeteners Negatively Regulate Pathogenic Characteristics of Two Model Gut Bacteria, E. coli and E. faecalis. International Journal of Molecular Sciences, 22(22), 5228. https:// doi.org/10.3390/ijms22105228

Skodje, G. I., et al. (2018). Fructan, Rather Than Gluten, Induces Symptoms in Patients With Self-Reported Non-Celiac Gluten Sensitivity. Gastroenterology, 154(3), 529-539.e2. https://doi.org/10.1053/j. gastro.2017.10.040

Suez, J., Cohen, Y., Valdés-Mas, R., Stein-Thoeringer, C. K., Segal, E., Elinav, E., et al. (2022). Personalized microbiome-driven effects of non-nutritive sweeteners on human glucose tolerance. Cell, 185(18), 3307-3328.e19. https://doi.org/10.1016/j.cell.2022.08.042

Takada, N., Nishida, K., Gondo, Y., Kikuchi-Hayakawa, H., Ishikawa, H., Suda, K., Kawai, M., Hoshi, R., Kuwano, Y., Miyazaki, K., & Rokutan, K. (2017). Beneficial effects of Lactobacillus casei strain Shirota on academic stress-induced sleep disturbance in healthy adults: A double-blind, randomized, placebo-controlled trial. Beneficial Microbes, 8(2), 153-162. https://doi. org/10.3920/BM2016.0069

Tarar, Z. I., Farooq, U., Zafar, Y., et al. (2023). Burden of anxiety and depression among hospitalized patients with irritable bowel syndrome:

A nationwide analysis. Irish Journal of Medical Science. Advance online publication. https://doi.org/10.1007/s11845-022-03258-6

Tillisch, K., Mayer, E. A., Gupta, A., Gill, Z., Brazeilles, R., Le Nevé, B., van Hylckama Vlieg, J. E. T., Guyonnet, D., Derrien, M., & Labus, J. S. (2017). Brain structure and response to emotional stimuli as related to gut microbial profiles in healthy women. Psychosomatic Medicine, 79(8), 905-913. https://doi.org/10.1097/PSY.0000000000000493

Tillisch, K., Labus, J., Kilpatrick, L., Jiang, Z., Stains, J., Ebrat, B., Guyonnet, D., Legrain-Raspaud, S., Trotin, B., Naliboff, B., & Mayer, E. A. (2013). Consumption of fermented milk product with probiotic modulates brain activity. Gastroenterology, 144(7), 1394-1401.e1-4. https://doi.org/10.1053/j.gastro.2013.02.043

Tsereteli, N., Vallat, R., Fernandez-Tajes, J., et al. (2022). Impact of insufficient sleep on dysregulated blood glucose control under standardized meal conditions. Diabetologia, 65, 356-365. https://doi.org/10.1007/s00125-021-05608-y

United Nations Food and Agriculture Organization. (1999). Women: Users, preservers and managers of agrobiodiversity. FAO.

Valdes, A. M., Walter, J., Segal, E., & Spector, T. D. (2018). Role of the gut microbiota in nutrition and health. BMJ, 361, k2179. https://doi.org/10.1136/bmj.k2179

Zhang, L., Reynolds Losin, E. A., Ashar, Y. K., Koban, L., & Wager, T. D. (2021). Gender biases in estimation of others' pain. The Journal of Pain, 22(9), 1048-1059.

Printed in Great Britain
by Amazon